VITALITY GUIDE TO ISOMETRIC EXERCISE FOR BACK PAIN

Natural Solutions for Back Pain Relief Through Safe Workouts

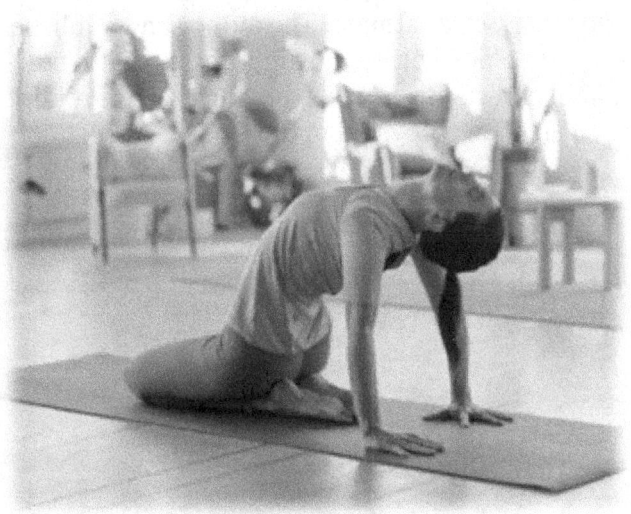

Caren Woods

Copyright © 2024 Caren Woods

All Rights Reserved

Disclaimer

Before beginning any exercise program, including the exercises described in this book, it is important to consult with your healthcare provider to ensure the activities are appropriate for your individual health and fitness level. The exercises and information provided in this book are for educational purposes only and should not be used as a substitute for professional medical advice, diagnosis, or treatment. The author and publisher are not responsible for any injuries or health issues that may result from following the exercise routines or suggestions provided in this book.

Table of Contents

VITALITY GUIDE TO ISOMETRIC EXERCISE FOR BACK PAIN i

Table of Contents iii

Introduction: Why This Book? How to Use This Book? 1

    The Importance of Back Health 2

    Why Isometric Exercises Work for Back Pain 6

    How to Use This Book for Maximum Benefit 11

Chapter 1: Understanding Back Pain and Isometric Exercises 15

    What is Back Pain? 17

    The Science Behind Isometric Exercises 22

    How Isometric Exercises Help Alleviate Back Pain 27

Chapter 2: Getting Started with Isometric Exercises 32

    Preparing Your Body: Warmups and Stretching 33

    Setting Realistic Goals for Your Back Health 38

    Safety Tips and Precautions 43

Chapter 3: Core Strength for a Healthy Back . 49

The Role of the Core in Back Pain Relief....50

Plank Variations: Building Core Stability...56

Bridge Hold: Strengthening the Lower Back 62

Chapter 4: Lower Body Strength for Spinal Support...68

Importance of Lower Body Strength for Back Health 69

Wall Sit: Targeting the Glutes and Quads...76

Glute Bridge: Enhancing Hip and Lower Back Strength 83

Chapter 5: Upper Body and Posture...............90

The Role of Upper Body Strength in Back Health..91

Wall Pushup: Engaging the Upper Body and Core...98

Shoulder Blade Squeeze: Improving Posture and Stability..103

Chapter 6: Flexibility and Mobility...............109

The Importance of Flexibility for Back Pain Relief..110

Cat-Cow Stretch: Spinal Mobility and Flexibility...116

Seated Forward Fold: Stretches for Hamstrings and Lower Back 123

Chapter 7: Functional Movements and Back Health 129

    The Connection Between Functional Movements and Back Health 130

    Standing Deadlift Hold: Strength and Balance 134

    BirdDog Hold: Core and Back Integration 139

Chapter 8: Advanced Isometric Exercises for Back Strength 144

    Advanced Plank Variations for Maximum Core Stability 145

    Wall Squat Hold: Increasing Endurance and Strength 150

    Superman Hold: Strengthening the Entire Back 154

Chapter 9: Nutrition and Hydration for Back Health 159

    Antiinflammatory Foods for Pain Relief ... 160

    The Importance of Calcium and Vitamin D for Bone Health 165

    Hydration: The Key to Muscle Function ... 170

Chapter 10: Putting It All Together 176

    Designing a Weekly Routine for Back Pain Relief 177

    Tracking Your Progress and Adjusting Your Routine 182

When to Seek Professional Help 187
Chapter 11: Maintaining Long Term Back Health 193
Preventing Future Back Pain 194
Staying Consistent with Your Exercises 198
Final Tips for a Healthy Spine 202
Conclusion 207

Introduction: Why This Book? How to Use This Book?

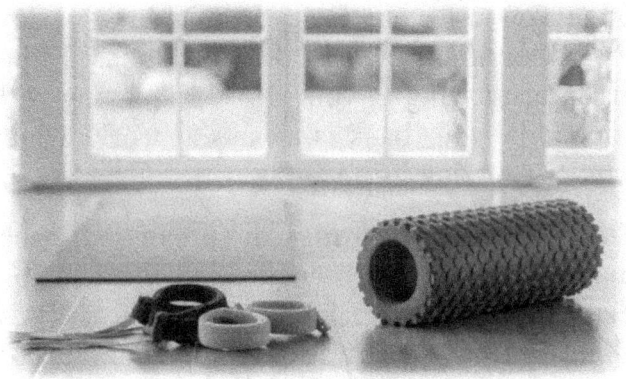

Isometric exercises involve holding your muscles in a fixed position without moving your joints, making them a gentle yet effective way to build strength. They are especially valuable for managing back pain, offering stability and relief without strain. With consistent practice, these exercises can help restore comfort and mobility to your daily life.

The Importance of Back Health

The health of your back affects more than just how comfortable you feel—it impacts your ability to live your life fully. Think about how often you use your back throughout the day. From bending down to tie your shoes, lifting groceries, sitting at your desk, or playing with your kids, your back is always at work. That's why prioritizing its health is critical.

Your spine is the central structure of your back, made up of 33 vertebrae cushioned by flexible discs that act as shock absorbers. These discs, along with your muscles, ligaments, and nerves, ensure stability and mobility. However, this intricate system is also delicate. Small disruptions, like weak muscles or poor posture, can trigger significant discomfort or even chronic pain.

Why Back Pain Is So Common

Back pain doesn't discriminate. It affects people of all ages and lifestyles. Common culprits include poor posture, sedentary habits, stress, and improper lifting techniques. Add in factors like aging, which can lead to wear and tear on your spine, or carrying extra weight that strains your lower back, and it's easy to see why so many people experience issues.

Even your mental health can play a role. Stress and anxiety often lead to muscle tension, which may amplify back discomfort. The bottom line is that your back is both strong and vulnerable. Treating it well helps prevent pain and ensures it can continue supporting you for years to come.

Why Your Back Deserves Attention Now

Sometimes, we only pay attention to our back when pain strikes. But that's like waiting for your car to break down before getting an oil change—it's far more effective to stay ahead of the problem. Regular care can prevent issues before they begin or keep existing discomfort from escalating.

A strong and healthy back improves your posture, enhances your mobility, and reduces your risk of injuries. Additionally, a well-supported spine contributes to better overall body mechanics, allowing your joints and muscles to work in harmony.

Practical Steps to Support Back Health

1. Posture Awareness

Start paying attention to how you sit, stand, and move. Keep your shoulders back, chest lifted, and spine in a neutral position.

2. Stay Active

Regular exercise, particularly activities that strengthen your core and back muscles, is vital.

3. Lift Smart

Use your legs, not your back, when lifting heavy objects. Bend at your knees and keep the load close to your body.

4. Use Ergonomics

Adjust your workspace to reduce strain. Ensure your chair supports your lower back and your computer is at eye level.

5. Maintain a Healthy Weight

Excess weight, especially around your abdomen, can strain your back. Focus on balanced eating habits and regular physical activity.

6. Stretch Often

Gentle stretching throughout the day helps maintain flexibility and prevents stiffness.

Even small adjustments to your routine can lead to significant improvements in your back health.

Strategic Suggestions

A healthy back doesn't just happen—it requires attention and care. Understand its importance and making thoughtful lifestyle choices, so you can protect it for the long term. Start with small, manageable changes today, and your back will thank you with improved comfort, strength, and resilience tomorrow.

Why Isometric Exercises Work for Back Pain

Back pain can make movement feel like a challenge, leaving you unsure about how to exercise safely. Isometric exercises offer a practical solution. They strengthen muscles without requiring complex movements, making them ideal for managing and preventing back pain. When your back hurts, the thought of exercising might feel intimidating. The fear of making the pain worse can lead you to avoid physical activity altogether. However, staying still for too long can weaken your muscles further, potentially worsening the problem. This is where isometric exercises step in as a safe and effective option for addressing back pain.

What Are Isometric Exercises?

Isometric exercises involve contracting your muscles without moving your joints. Think of holding a plank or pushing your hands together in front of your chest. These exercises build strength and endurance by engaging muscles in a static position, which is particularly helpful if moving causes discomfort.

For your back, isometric exercises can target the muscles that support your spine, including the core, lower back, and surrounding stabilizers. Strengthen these areas to create a sturdy framework that helps reduce pain and prevents future injuries.

Why They're Perfect for Back Pain

There are several reasons why isometric exercises are well-suited for back pain relief:

1. Low Impact

Since these exercises don't involve sudden or repetitive movements, they put minimal stress on your joints and spine. This makes them an excellent choice for people with sensitive or injured backs.

2. Muscle Activation

Isometric exercises effectively engage deep stabilizing muscles that traditional workouts might miss. Strengthening these muscles can improve spinal alignment and reduce strain.

3. Control and Safety

Unlike dynamic exercises, which require movement, isometric exercises give you more control over the intensity and duration. This reduces the risk of aggravating existing pain.

4. Improved Stability

A stronger core and back mean better support for your spine, reducing the likelihood of future injuries.

5. Adaptability

These exercises are easily modified to suit different fitness levels, so you can start small and gradually progress as your strength improves.

Examples of Isometric Exercises for Back Pain

Here are a few beginner-friendly isometric exercises that can help ease back pain. Remember to breathe deeply and focus on maintaining good form throughout each exercise:

1. Wall Sit

- Stand with your back against a wall and your feet about two feet away from it.
- Slowly slide down the wall until your knees are bent at a 90-degree angle, as if sitting in an invisible chair.
- Hold this position for 10–30 seconds, engaging your core and keeping your back flat against the wall.

2. Plank

- Lie face down on the floor, then lift yourself onto your forearms and toes, forming a straight line from head to heels.

- Keep your core tight and avoid letting your hips sag or rise too high.
- Hold for 10–30 seconds, gradually increasing the duration as you build strength.

3. Bridge Hold

- Lie on your back with your knees bent and feet flat on the ground.
- Press your heels into the floor and lift your hips until your body forms a straight line from your shoulders to your knees.
- Squeeze your glutes and hold for 10–20 seconds before lowering back down.

4. Seated Ab Squeeze

- Sit upright in a chair with your feet flat on the floor.
- Place your hands on your thighs and press down gently as you engage your abdominal muscles.
- Hold the contraction for 10–15 seconds, then release and repeat.

5. Side Plank

- Lie on your side with your legs straight and your elbow directly under your shoulder.

- Lift your hips off the ground, forming a straight line from head to heels.
- Hold for 10–20 seconds, then switch sides.

How to Incorporate These Exercises

To see results, consistency is key. Aim to perform isometric exercises 3–4 times per week. Start with shorter hold times and fewer repetitions, gradually increasing as your strength improves. If you're unsure about proper technique, consulting a physical therapist or trainer can help you get started safely.

Strategic Suggestions

Isometric exercises offer a simple, effective way to strengthen your back and manage pain without risking further strain. Incorporate them into your routine regularly, and you'll build a solid foundation of strength and stability. With time and consistency, these exercises can help you move through life more comfortably and confidently.

How to Use This Book for Maximum Benefit

A resource is only as valuable as how well you use it. This book is designed to guide you in overcoming back pain with simple, practical isometric exercises. To achieve the best results, you'll need a clear understanding of how to approach it. Taking on a book about managing back pain can feel like embarking on a big project. But don't worry—this guide is meant to be user-friendly and actionable.

To make the most of it, you'll want to take things step by step and adapt the advice to your unique needs. Here's how to ensure this book becomes your trusted companion on the path to a healthier back.

Understand the Structure

This book is organized to provide a balanced mix of education and actionable steps. The introduction lays out why back health matters and why isometric exercises are a good fit for managing pain. We will dive into specific exercises, tips, and strategies to help you gradually build strength and reduce discomfort.

Familiarize yourself with the layout so you know where to find key information. If you're experiencing acute back pain, start with gentler exercises outlined in the early sections. If you're further along in your recovery or prevention efforts, you might find the more advanced exercises and tips helpful.

Commit to Consistency

Consistency is one of the most important factors for success. You won't see results from just trying an exercise once or twice. Make it a point to carve out time for these activities regularly, daily or several times a week. Think of this book as a roadmap. Each section builds on the last, so sticking with the program is crucial.

To make things easier, integrate these exercises into your routine. Perhaps you can start your day with a quick session or use them as a midday break from work. The key is to treat them as a non-negotiable part of your schedule.

Follow Instructions Carefully

The exercises described in this book are most effective when done correctly. Pay close attention to the detailed instructions for each move. Even a small error in form can reduce the effectiveness of an exercise or, worse, exacerbate your discomfort.

Take your time learning each position. If a movement feels unfamiliar or challenging, don't rush through it. Instead, focus on mastering the basics before progressing to more advanced variations.

Personalize Your Approach

Back pain isn't a one-size-fits-all issue. The strategies in this book are designed to be flexible and adaptable to different needs. If you have a pre-existing condition or a specific type of back pain, you may need to adjust some exercises to suit your situation.

For example, if holding a plank feels too intense at first, you can modify it by lowering your knees to the floor. Similarly, if you're feeling particularly stiff one day, focus on lighter stretches and shorter hold times.

Track Your Progress

One of the best ways to stay motivated is to track your improvements. Consider keeping a journal where you record which exercises you've done, how long you held each position, and how your back feels afterward.

Over time, you'll likely notice that you can hold positions longer or that certain exercises feel easier.

Practice Patience and Self-Care

While this book offers effective tools for managing back pain, remember that healing and strengthening take time. Avoid the temptation to push yourself too hard or skip ahead to more advanced exercises before you're ready.

Also, listen to your body. If an exercise feels painful or uncomfortable, stop and reassess. It's normal to feel some muscle activation during these movements, but sharp pain is a sign to ease up or consult a healthcare professional.

Leverage the Supportive Resources

In addition to the exercises, this book includes tips on posture, ergonomics, and lifestyle adjustments. Don't overlook these sections—they can greatly enhance the effectiveness of your practice. Small changes in how you sit, stand, or lift objects can complement the strength you're building through isometric exercises.

Strategic Suggestions

Using this book effectively means more than just reading—it's about creating a routine and staying consistent. Tailor the exercises to your needs, track your progress, and approach the program with patience. With commitment and thoughtful effort, you'll find yourself on the path to stronger, pain-free days. Now, take the first step!

Chapter 1: Understanding Back Pain and Isometric Exercises

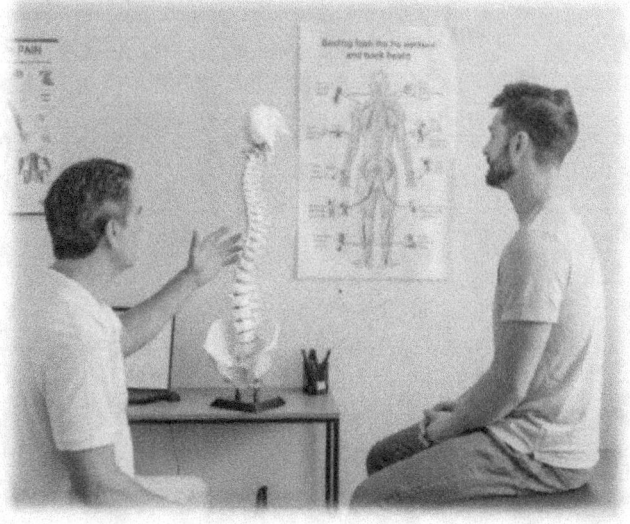

Back pain is a physical discomfort that affects daily life and mobility, often caused by strain, posture issues, or underlying conditions. Understanding its causes is essential for effective relief. Pairing this knowledge with isometric exercises, a proven method to strengthen and stabilize muscles, can offer significant benefits for your back health.

What is Back Pain?

Back pain is a common issue that can affect anyone, regardless of age or lifestyle. It refers to discomfort or stiffness in the back, often caused by strain, poor posture, or underlying health conditions. Understanding what triggers back pain and its impact is the first step toward managing and preventing it effectively.

Back pain is one of the most widespread physical complaints. You've likely experienced it at some point—a twinge after bending awkwardly, stiffness from sitting too long, or a sharp ache after lifting something heavy. While it's easy to shrug off as an annoyance, back pain can significantly affect your quality of life if left unchecked.

Types of Back Pain

Back pain isn't a one-size-fits-all issue. It can be acute, lasting a few days to weeks, or chronic, persisting for months or even years. Identifying the type of pain you're experiencing helps in choosing the right approach to manage it.

1. Acute Back Pain

This usually comes on suddenly and is often linked to a specific event, like lifting something heavy or a sudden awkward movement. It can be sharp and severe but typically improves within a few weeks with rest and proper care.

2. Chronic Back Pain

This lasts longer than 12 weeks and can persist even after the original injury or strain has healed. Chronic pain is often linked to ongoing conditions like arthritis or disc problems.

Back pain can also vary in location; Upper Back Pain or Lower Back Pain.

Common Causes of Back Pain

Understanding what causes back pain can empower you to make changes that protect your back. Here are some of the most common culprits:

1. Poor Posture

Slouching or hunching over, especially for long hours at a desk, can strain your back muscles.

2. Sedentary Lifestyle

Lack of movement can weaken your back and core muscles, making your spine less supported.

3. Overuse or Strain

Overdoing physical activities or lifting heavy objects improperly can lead to strained muscles.

4. Age-Related Changes

As you get older, the discs in your spine can degenerate, leading to conditions like arthritis or spinal stenosis.

5. Stress and Tension

Emotional stress can cause muscle tension, especially in the neck and back.

6. Underlying Conditions

Herniated discs, sciatica, and osteoporosis can all contribute to chronic back pain.

Why Back Pain Matters

Your back plays a central role in your body's overall function. It supports your weight, allows movement, and protects your spinal cord, which is essential for nerve function. When pain strikes, it doesn't just make daily tasks harder—it can affect your mood, sleep, and even mental health.

Ignoring back pain often leads to compensatory habits, like leaning more on one side or avoiding movement altogether. These can create a vicious cycle of worsening pain and reduced mobility. Addressing the root cause is key to breaking this cycle.

Signs You Shouldn't Ignore

While most back pain is manageable with lifestyle adjustments, some symptoms warrant medical attention:

- Pain that radiates down one or both legs, possibly indicating sciatica.
- Numbness or tingling, which could signal nerve involvement.
- Pain following an injury, such as a fall or accident.
- Loss of bladder or bowel control, a rare but serious symptom requiring immediate care.

The Good News: Back Pain Can Be Managed

Most back pain doesn't require surgery or invasive treatments. Often, a combination of movement, strength-building, and lifestyle adjustments can make a huge difference. That's where isometric exercises come into play. Unlike dynamic movements, they help strengthen the muscles supporting your back without adding strain.

Tips for Easing Back Pain

1. Stay Active

Gentle activities like walking or stretching can prevent stiffness.

2. Mind Your Posture

Sit and stand with your shoulders back and your spine in a neutral position.

3. Strengthen Core Muscles

A strong core reduces the load on your back.

4. Use Proper Lifting Techniques

Bend at your knees, not your waist, when picking up heavy objects.

5. Prioritize Rest and Recovery

If you've strained your back, allow time to heal but avoid prolonged inactivity.

Strategic Suggestions

Back pain may be common, but it doesn't have to be a permanent fixture in your life. Recognizing its causes and impact is your first step toward relief. With knowledge and practical tools, you can protect your back, regain comfort, and stay active without fear of recurring pain. Take control today.

The Science Behind Isometric Exercises

Isometric exercises are unique in how they engage your muscles without requiring movement. They activate and strengthen specific muscle groups by holding positions, making them effective for building stability. When you think of exercise, you might picture dynamic movements like running, lifting weights, or yoga poses. Isometric exercises, however, are different—they involve holding a position rather than moving through a range of motion.

What Happens During Isometric Exercises?

In isometric exercises, your muscles contract without shortening or lengthening. For instance, when you hold a plank, your abdominal, back, and shoulder muscles are all working hard to stabilize your body, even though you're not moving.

This static contraction engages muscle fibers and increases tension, which strengthens the targeted muscles over time. Unlike dynamic exercises, which rely on repetitive motion, isometric exercises allow you to build strength without putting additional strain on your joints or spine.

How Isometric Exercises Benefit Your Back

Weak or imbalanced muscles can lead to poor posture and pain. Isometric exercises specifically target these stabilizing muscles, helping to:

1. Improve Stability

Your back relies on a network of muscles to stay aligned and stable. Isometric exercises like planks or wall sits strengthen these muscles, making your spine less vulnerable to strain or injury.

2. Reduce Stress on Joints

Since isometric exercises don't involve movement, they're gentle on your joints, making them ideal for people with back pain or limited mobility.

3. Enhance Muscle Endurance

Holding static positions builds the endurance of stabilizing muscles, helping them better support your back during everyday activities.

4. Promote Better Posture

Strengthening the muscles around your spine naturally encourages proper posture, which reduces pressure on your lower back.

The Role of Core and Stabilizer Muscles

Your core muscles—those around your abdomen, back, and pelvis—play a critical role in supporting your spine. When these muscles are strong, they act as a natural corset, keeping your back aligned and reducing the risk of pain.

Isometric exercises are particularly effective at engaging the deep core muscles, such as the transverse abdominis, which often go unnoticed during dynamic workouts. These muscles provide a stable foundation for your spine and improve your overall balance and coordination.

How Isometric Exercises Improve Blood Flow

When you hold an isometric position, the sustained muscle contraction temporarily reduces blood flow to the area. Once you release the position, blood rushes back into the muscles, delivering oxygen and nutrients. This process can help reduce inflammation and promote healing in areas affected by pain or stiffness.

Why Isometric Exercises Are Safe for Back Pain

Unlike high-impact activities that can jolt your spine or cause overextension, isometric exercises allow you to control the level of intensity. You can start with shorter hold times and gradually increase as your strength improves, minimizing the risk of overexertion.

Additionally, isometric exercises can be adapted to suit your fitness level. For example, if a traditional plank feels too challenging, you can modify it by lowering your knees to the floor. This flexibility makes them accessible to people of all abilities.

Scientific Evidence Supporting Isometric Exercises

Research highlights the effectiveness of isometric exercises for pain management and muscle strengthening. Studies have shown that:

1. Improved Muscle Strength

Isometric training can increase strength by targeting specific muscle groups without additional strain.

2. Pain Reduction

Regular practice of isometric exercises has been linked to reduced pain in conditions like chronic lower back pain.

3. Postural Improvements

Strengthening stabilizer muscles with isometric holds leads to better posture, which can alleviate pressure on the spine.

Examples of Back-Friendly Isometric Exercises

Here are some isometric exercises to strengthen your back safely:

- **Plank:** Activates your core and supports your spine.
- **Wall Sit:** Strengthens lower back and leg muscles.
- **Bridge Hold:** Targets glutes and lower back stabilizers.
- **Side Plank:** Engages oblique muscles and improves lateral stability.

Strategic Suggestions

The science behind isometric exercises highlights their effectiveness in strengthening stabilizing muscles and managing pain. These exercises build stability, improve blood flow, and reduce strain on your spine. Incorporate them into your routine to enhance your back health safely and steadily, setting the stage for lasting relief and strength.

How Isometric Exercises Help Alleviate Back Pain

Back pain can feel overwhelming, but isometric exercises offer a practical and gentle solution. They strengthen muscles, improve stability, and reduce strain on your spine, making them ideal for managing discomfort. When dealing with back pain, you may feel unsure about which exercises are safe or effective. Isometric exercises stand out because they build strength without requiring repetitive movement, which can sometimes worsen discomfort. Instead of adding strain, they provide targeted support to the muscles that need it most.

Strengthening Key Support Muscles

One of the main reasons isometric exercises are effective is their ability to engage stabilizing muscles. These are the muscles around your spine, hips, and core that work together to support your back.

For example, holding a plank position activates your transverse abdominis, a deep core muscle crucial for spine stability. Similarly, exercises like wall sits or bridge holds strengthen the glutes and lower back muscles, reducing the load on your spine. Fortify these muscles to essentially build a protective layer for your back.

Reducing Load on the Spine

Back pain often results from too much stress on your spinal discs or vertebrae. Weak muscles around the spine force it to take on more pressure, leading to discomfort or injury. Isometric exercises help redistribute this load.

When you practice isometric holds, your muscles take on the task of stabilization, relieving pressure on your spine. For example, a side plank strengthens your oblique muscles, which support the sides of your lower back and reduce strain on your lumbar spine.

Improving Posture

Poor posture is a common cause of back pain, especially for people who spend long hours sitting or standing. Isometric exercises naturally encourage better posture by targeting the muscles that keep your spine aligned.

Take the wall sit as an example. Hold this position, so you're not only strengthening your thighs and lower back but also training your body to maintain a neutral spine.

Increasing Blood Flow and Reducing Inflammation

When you perform an isometric exercise, the sustained muscle contraction promotes blood flow to the area once the hold is released. This increased circulation helps deliver oxygen and nutrients to your back muscles, aiding recovery and reducing inflammation.

Inflammation is a common culprit behind back pain, especially in conditions like sciatica or arthritis. Regular isometric practice can help manage this inflammation, providing relief over time.

Easing Muscle Tension and Stress

Stress and tension often manifest in the back, leading to tightness and discomfort. Isometric exercises help ease this tension through controlled engagement and release of muscles.

For instance, holding a gentle bridge position can stretch and activate your lower back, relieving tightness. Similarly, a plank hold activates your core muscles, encouraging your back to relax and release built-up tension.

Customizable Intensity

Another advantage of isometric exercises is their adaptability. You can adjust the difficulty level based on your pain and fitness level. If an exercise feels too intense, you can modify it by shortening the hold time or using props for support.

For example, if a traditional plank feels challenging, try performing it with your knees on the floor. As your strength improves, you can progress to the full version. This customization ensures you're working at a safe intensity that benefits your back without risking further strain.

Boosting Confidence and Mobility

Living with back pain can make you hesitant to move, fearing that activity might worsen your condition. Isometric exercises are a gentle way to regain confidence in your body's abilities.

These exercises help you feel stronger and more in control, which can encourage you to stay active. Over time, this improved mobility can reduce stiffness and make everyday movements—like bending or lifting—less daunting.

Examples of Back-Friendly Isometric Exercises

Here are a few isometric exercises to include in your routine:

- **Plank Hold:** Strengthens your core and supports your spine.
- **Wall Sit:** Builds strength in your lower back and legs.
- **Side Plank:** Enhances lateral stability and engages obliques.

- **Bridge Hold:** Activates your glutes and lower back.

Practice these exercises regularly, aiming for 20–30 seconds per hold to start. Gradually increase the duration as your strength improves.

Strategic Suggestions

Isometric exercises offer a safe, effective way to relieve back pain. They strengthen key muscles, improve posture, and reduce strain on your spine. With consistency and patience, these exercises can help you regain mobility and confidence, setting the stage for a healthier, pain-free back. Start with small steps and build from there.

Chapter 2: Getting Started with Isometric Exercises

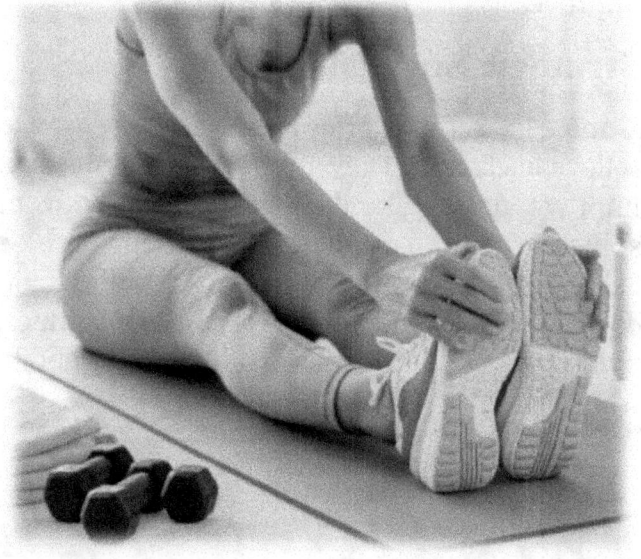

Isometric exercises involve holding a position to engage and strengthen muscles without movement. This type of exercise is crucial for building stability and improving strength, especially for managing back pain. Getting started with these exercises can help you safely strengthen your muscles, relieve discomfort, and support long-term back health.

Preparing Your Body: Warmups and Stretching

Warming up and stretching are key to preparing your body for exercise and preventing injury. Before starting isometric exercises, it's essential to properly activate and loosen up your muscles, especially in your back and core. This helps enhance performance, improve flexibility, and protect your body from unnecessary strain.

When it comes to isometric exercises, the goal is to strengthen your muscles while maintaining stability and control. Warming up and stretching are important steps in preparing your muscles, joints, and tissues for the work ahead. Let's break down how to effectively warm up and stretch before you start your isometric exercises.

Why Warmup Matters

A good warm-up helps increase blood flow to your muscles, making them more flexible and ready for action. When you warm up, you're essentially telling your muscles that they need to be active. This helps to prevent stiffness and reduces the likelihood of injury. A proper warm-up can also improve your performance by activating the muscles you'll be using during your workout, ensuring they're engaged and ready to work.

For isometric exercises, this is particularly important. These exercises involve holding positions that put sustained tension on certain muscles, like your core, glutes, or back. If those muscles aren't warmed up, they could fatigue too quickly or become strained.

What Should a Good Warm-Up Include?

The warm-up should be light and dynamic, not static. This means you should focus on movements that get your heart rate up and increase blood flow to the muscles, rather than holding positions for extended periods. Aim for about 5-10 minutes of activity. Here are a few examples of warm-up activities that will benefit your back and core:

1. Gentle Cardio (5 minutes)

Start with a low-impact activity like walking or marching in place. This helps raise your body temperature and improves circulation to your muscles. If you prefer, you can try cycling on a stationary bike or a gentle jog to gradually increase your heart rate.

2. Torso Twists

Stand with your feet hip-width apart, and twist your torso from side to side gently. This warms up your spine and helps increase flexibility in your back and core.

3. Hip Circles

Stand with your feet a little wider than hip-width, place your hands on your hips, and slowly rotate your hips in circles—first clockwise, then counterclockwise. This helps to loosen up your lower back and hips.

4. Leg Swings

While holding onto a wall or chair for balance, swing one leg forward and backward, then side to side. This dynamic movement stretches your hip flexors and hamstrings, improving lower body flexibility and stability.

Stretching: Enhancing Flexibility

Stretching helps lengthen your muscles and increase flexibility, which can improve your range of motion and prevent injury. Before engaging in isometric exercises, incorporating stretches can also help relax tight muscles and increase your mobility. Stretching is particularly important for your back, hips, and legs—areas that play a crucial role in supporting your spine and posture.

When stretching before isometric exercises, focus on dynamic stretches, which involve movement rather than holding a position. Static stretching, where you hold a stretch for an extended period, is best reserved for the cool-down period after your workout. Dynamic stretches allow your muscles to lengthen and prepare for the controlled tension of isometric holds.

Essential Stretches for Your Back and Core

Here are a few stretches that can help you prepare your body for isometric exercises, particularly focusing on your back and core muscles:

1. Cat-Cow Stretch

Start on your hands and knees in a tabletop position. On an inhale, arch your back and drop your belly toward the floor (Cow Pose). On an exhale, round your spine and tuck your chin (Cat Pose). This stretches the spine and activates the core, promoting flexibility and range of motion.

2. Downward-Facing Dog

From a tabletop position, lift your hips toward the ceiling, creating an inverted V shape with your body. This stretch targets your hamstrings, back, and shoulders, improving flexibility and elongating the spine.

3. Standing Forward Fold

Stand tall with your feet hip-width apart. Slowly bend forward at the hips, keeping your knees soft. Reach for the floor, allowing your head and neck to relax. This stretches your hamstrings, lower back, and calves.

4. Pelvic Tilts

Lie on your back with your knees bent and feet flat on the floor. Tighten your abdominal muscles and gently tilt your pelvis upward, pressing your lower back into the floor. This movement helps activate your core and stretch your lower back.

Cooling Down After Your Warm-Up

Once you've completed your warm-up and stretching, it's time to prepare for the isometric exercises. A short cooldown after your warm-up, involving deep breathing and gentle stretches, can help lower your heart rate and relax your muscles. Doing so will ensure you're physically and mentally ready to perform the isometric holds.

Strategic Suggestions

Warming up and stretching are vital steps to ensure that your body is properly prepared for isometric exercises. Engage in light cardio, dynamic stretches, and targeted flexibility work to enhance muscle readiness, reduce risk of injury, and optimize performance. Incorporating these habits into your routine will improve your results and overall safety.

Setting Realistic Goals for Your Back Health

Setting realistic goals is an essential part of improving your back health. It helps keep you motivated, track your progress, and ensure that your efforts align with your personal needs and abilities. When it comes to improving your back health, one of the most important steps is setting realistic and attainable goals. Without clear goals, you might find yourself frustrated, unsure of your progress, or even tempted to give up.

Why Setting Goals Matters

Goals give you direction. They break down the long-term process of improving your back health into smaller, manageable steps. This structured approach prevents overwhelm and helps you see tangible progress, which is essential for staying on track. Without a specific target, it can be easy to fall into a routine without noticing significant results. Set realistic goals to ensure that you are actively working toward better back health each day.

Types of Goals to Set for Back Health

When setting goals, it's important to make them specific, measurable, achievable, relevant, and time-bound—often referred to as SMART goals. This structure helps ensure that your goals are clear, actionable, and trackable. Let's break down different types of goals that can help with back health.

Strengthening Goals

Strengthening your back and core muscles is a primary focus when it comes to managing back pain. You can set specific goals to gradually build strength through isometric exercises. For example, you might aim to hold a plank for 20 seconds without pain, then gradually work up to 60 seconds over a few weeks.

Another strengthening goal could involve targeting specific muscles that support your spine. For instance, strengthening your glutes, lower back, and abdominal muscles can provide stability and reduce strain on your spine. You could set a goal to complete three sets of a specific exercise, such as the bridge hold or side plank, with proper form and control.

Flexibility Goals

Tight muscles often contribute to back pain. Stretching and improving flexibility can help alleviate tension and improve your range of motion. A flexibility goal might be to improve the length of time you can hold stretches like the forward fold or cat-cow, or to gradually work toward deeper stretches as your flexibility increases.

For example, if you're currently unable to touch your toes, a realistic flexibility goal might be to reach your knees first, then gradually work down to your shins and eventually your toes. This not only helps with back pain but also supports overall mobility and flexibility, which is crucial for long-term spinal health.

Pain Reduction Goals

If you're managing chronic back pain, one of your most important goals might be to reduce the frequency or intensity of pain. Start by tracking your pain levels daily and setting specific targets. For example, you might set a goal to reduce pain by a certain number of points on a 10-point scale over the course of a few weeks.

You can achieve this goal by incorporating isometric exercises into your routine to build strength and stability, which can help alleviate discomfort. As your muscles become stronger and your posture improves, you may notice a decrease in pain and greater mobility.

Posture and Alignment Goals

Improving your posture is essential for long-term back health. If you spend a lot of time sitting, especially at a desk or in front of a computer, poor posture can contribute to back pain. Setting a goal to improve your posture is a step toward reducing strain on your spine.

A posture-related goal might be to check your posture every 30 minutes throughout the day or to consciously engage your core muscles while sitting. You could also aim to incorporate back-strengthening exercises, such as the plank or wall sit, to promote better posture and spinal alignment.

Consistency and Routine Goals

Consistency is key when it comes to back health. Setting goals for how often you'll practice your isometric exercises and stretching can ensure that you stay on track. For example, you might set a goal to complete a 15-minute stretching session three times a week or to hold a plank for 30 seconds every morning.

Tracking these small, consistent actions over time helps you build a routine and steadily progress toward your larger goals. Establishing a regular routine can make back-strengthening exercises a habit, which will support long-term relief and better overall health.

How to Stay Motivated and Adjust Your Goals

It's important to stay motivated throughout the process. As you achieve one goal, set a new one to keep moving forward. Remember, progress may be slow at times, but it's crucial to celebrate each milestone along the way. Don't be discouraged if things don't go as planned; setbacks are normal, and adjusting your goals is part of the process.

If you're experiencing setbacks in your pain levels or progress, consider adjusting the difficulty of your exercises or stretching routine. You might want to modify your goals based on your current abilities, or consult a healthcare professional for additional guidance. The key is to make steady progress at a pace that works for your body.

Strategic Suggestions

Setting realistic goals for your back health is crucial for staying on track and motivated. Regardless of if your goals focus on strength, flexibility, pain reduction, or posture, they provide clear direction and measurable progress. Consistency and small adjustments will keep you moving forward and ultimately lead to better back health.

Safety Tips and Precautions

Isometric exercises are a powerful tool for improving back health, but performing them incorrectly or without proper precautions can lead to injury. Safety should always be your priority. Isometric exercises are a great way to strengthen your back and reduce pain, but as with any form of exercise, it's important to approach them with caution. Without proper form and safety measures, you could risk straining muscles, overstretching, or aggravating existing back pain. The key to success with isometric exercises is to listen to your body and follow guidelines that protect your spine, joints, and muscles.

Let's explore the most important safety tips and precautions to ensure that your workout is both effective and safe.

1. Start Slow and Gradual Progression

One of the most important safety tips is to start slowly and progress at your own pace. Isometric exercises are designed to build strength over time, and attempting to push yourself too quickly can lead to strain or injury. For beginners, start with basic exercises that involve less intensity or shorter hold times.

Begin with just a few seconds of holding a position (like a plank or wall sit) and gradually increase the duration as you feel more comfortable. It's always better to start on the lower end and work your way up rather than risk overexertion. A good rule of thumb is to increase the hold time or intensity by just a few seconds every week until you build the necessary strength and endurance.

2. Maintain Proper Form

Form is everything when it comes to isometric exercises. Poor form can lead to unnecessary pressure on your spine and muscles, leading to discomfort or injury. Always ensure that your posture and alignment are correct throughout each exercise.

For example, when performing a plank, make sure your body is in a straight line from head to heels. Avoid letting your lower back sag or your hips rise too high. If you feel your form slipping, take a break or shorten the hold time to prevent strain.

3. Engage Your Core and Focus on Breathing

Proper breathing is essential during isometric exercises. Holding your breath while attempting a hold can lead to increased pressure on your back and abdomen, which may increase your risk of injury. Instead, focus on steady, deep breathing.

Engaging your core muscles throughout the exercise also ensures that your spine is properly supported. Your core should be actively engaged, but you shouldn't hold your breath to tighten it. Breathe in deeply through your nose and out through your mouth while keeping your stomach muscles active and stable.

4. Know When to Stop

Your body will always give you signals if something isn't right. It's important to stop immediately if you experience any sharp or sudden pain, dizziness, or discomfort. These sensations may indicate that you're pushing too hard or straining an area of your body.

When you're just starting with isometric exercises, it's normal to feel muscle fatigue or mild soreness, but sharp pain is never a good sign. Trust your body and take a break if you feel anything that's not typical muscle burn or fatigue. Rest is an important part of your workout routine, and it's better to be cautious than risk an injury that could set you back.

5. Use Proper Equipment

While isometric exercises generally don't require equipment, certain props like yoga mats, stability balls, or resistance bands can make exercises more effective and comfortable. Using a soft, non-slip mat for exercises like planks or wall sits will ensure you have adequate support.

If you're using resistance bands, be sure to choose the correct resistance level for your current strength. Over-stretching or using too much resistance can put undue strain on your back. Additionally, avoid using any equipment that feels unstable or uncomfortable during the exercises. Comfort and stability are key for maintaining safety and proper form.

6. Stay Consistent but Avoid Overtraining

Consistency is important when it comes to strengthening your back, but overtraining can be harmful. Your muscles need time to recover and rebuild after each workout, so be mindful of how often you're performing isometric exercises.

Ideally, aim to perform isometric exercises 2-3 times per week with at least a day of rest in between. This allows your muscles to rest, which helps prevent overuse injuries like muscle strain or joint irritation. Make sure you're also including other forms of movement in your routine, like walking or swimming, to promote overall body health and flexibility.

7. Listen to Your Body and Modify as Needed

It's important to stay tuned in to how your body is feeling during and after isometric exercises. If you experience discomfort in your back, knees, or hips, make modifications to the exercises to reduce strain.

For example, if you're performing a wall sit and feel pressure on your knees, adjust your leg position so your knees are at a more comfortable angle. Similarly, if you're holding a plank and your lower back is aching, reduce the hold time or try a modified version of the exercise, such as performing it from your knees.

8. Consult a Professional if Needed

If you're new to isometric exercises or experiencing ongoing back pain, consider consulting with a healthcare professional, such as a physical therapist or chiropractor. They can assess your individual condition, help you with proper form, and recommend modifications to suit your specific needs.

Strategic Suggestions

Safety is key when starting isometric exercises for back pain. Progress slowly, maintain proper form, and listen to your body, so you can minimize the risk of injury while maximizing the benefits of your workout. Consistency, patience, and attention to safety will help you achieve long-term back health and strength.

Chapter 3: Core Strength for a Healthy Back

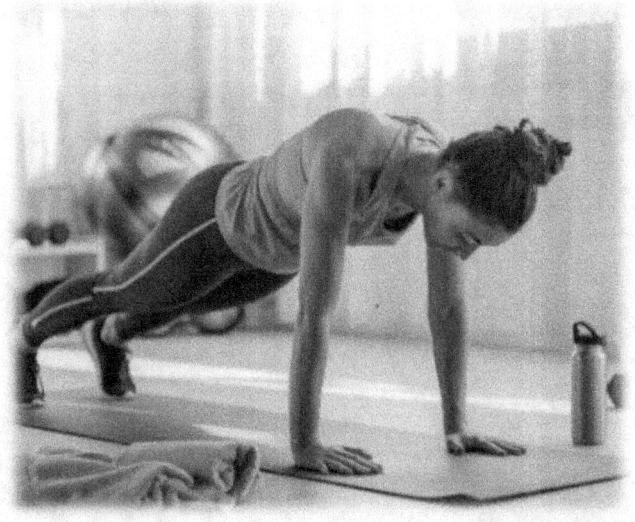

Core strength refers to the ability to engage and control the muscles in your abdomen, lower back, and pelvis. A strong core is essential for supporting your spine, maintaining proper posture, and preventing back pain. Strengthening these muscles helps improve stability, reduce discomfort, and promote long-term back health.

The Role of the Core in Back Pain Relief

Your core is more than just your abs—it's a complex system of muscles that support your spine and help you move without pain. Strengthening your core is one of the most effective ways to reduce back pain. Your core plays a critical role in the overall health of your back. It's not just about having toned abs; the core encompasses a variety of muscles, including the muscles in your abdomen, lower back, hips, and pelvis. These muscles work together to support your spine, protect it from injury, and help you maintain balance and proper posture. When your core is weak or imbalanced, it can lead to back pain, discomfort, and even injury.

Let's dive into how strengthening your core can alleviate and prevent back pain, and why it's such a crucial part of any back pain relief strategy.

1. The Core and Its Connection to the Spine

Your spine is a complex structure made up of vertebrae, discs, nerves, and muscles. Without sufficient support, the spine can become misaligned, leading to pain and discomfort. The muscles of your core are responsible for stabilizing the spine and providing it with the support it needs to function properly.

When your core muscles are weak, your back muscles have to compensate, often leading to strain and tension. This can result in poor posture, spinal misalignment, and increased pressure on the discs in your lower back, which can lead to herniated discs or sciatica. Strengthening the muscles of your core helps relieve this pressure, protect the spine, and reduce the risk of back pain.

2. Preventing Back Pain Through Stability

One of the main roles of the core muscles is to maintain stability in the spine. Stability refers to your body's ability to control movement and resist forces that could disrupt the alignment of your spine. A strong core can help prevent back pain by providing stability during everyday movements, such as sitting, standing, bending, and lifting.

When you engage your core muscles, you create a natural "brace" around your spine, protecting it from sudden jerks, twists, or heavy lifting. This is particularly helpful when you're lifting objects, such as something as simple as a grocery bag or as heavy as a box. If your core is weak, the risk of straining your back during lifting is much higher.

Think of your core as a sturdy foundation—just like a building needs a solid base to stay upright, your spine needs a strong core to stay in alignment and avoid injury.

3. The Core as a Support System for Posture

Good posture is essential for reducing back pain, and your core plays a huge role in maintaining that posture. When your core muscles are weak, it's easy to slouch or lean forward, which puts extra pressure on your lower back and can lead to discomfort over time. Strong core muscles, however, help you maintain an upright posture, keeping your spine properly aligned and reducing strain on the muscles and discs of the back.

Poor posture is often the result of imbalances in the muscles that support the spine. If certain muscles, such as your core or back muscles, are weak, other muscles, like those in your hips and shoulders, may take over, leading to discomfort and pain. Strengthening your core muscles helps to correct these imbalances, ensuring that your spine stays in a neutral, healthy position.

4. Reducing the Risk of Injury

When your core is strong, it reduces the risk of injury in both everyday activities and exercise.

For instance, when you twist, bend, or reach for something, your core acts as a protective barrier for your spine. Without adequate core strength, your body compensates, leading to poor mechanics, muscle strain, and back pain.

Core strengthening exercises, like isometric holds, help teach your body how to engage and protect your spine during movement. This protective mechanism reduces the likelihood of acute injuries, such as sprains or strains, and helps your muscles function more efficiently.

5. Improving Flexibility and Mobility

A well-developed core also improves flexibility and mobility in your back and hips. When your core is strong, it allows your spine and surrounding muscles to move more freely, without restriction. This is important not just for preventing back pain, but also for maintaining overall mobility as you age.

Isometric exercises, such as planks and bridges, help engage both your deep and superficial core muscles. This engagement helps you maintain control over your body's movement, which is essential for flexibility and mobility. As you work to strengthen your core, you'll notice that you can move with greater ease and comfort, with less stiffness in your back.

6. Incorporating Core Strength into Daily Life

While targeted exercises are important for building core strength, you can also engage your core throughout the day to help support your back. For example, when sitting at your desk or standing, make a conscious effort to engage your abdominal muscles and maintain a neutral spine.

This practice of "core engagement" can be done anytime, such as while you're walking, lifting, or even sitting. Training your core to engage naturally will help keep your back protected during everyday movements and reduce the likelihood of pain.

Conclusion

Core strength is essential for maintaining a healthy back and preventing back pain. When your core muscles are strong, your spine stays protected, your posture improves, and your risk of injury decreases. Building core strength through isometric exercises is one of the most effective ways to support your back and enjoy a pain-free lifestyle.

Strategic Suggestions

To reduce back pain, prioritize building core strength. Engage in regular core-strengthening exercises to improve your posture, stability, and flexibility, making your back more resilient to strain. Strengthening your core muscles not only helps protect your spine but also promotes better movement and overall well-being.

Plank Variations: Building Core Stability

The plank is one of the most effective exercises for strengthening your core and improving stability, especially for back health. Hold your body in a rigid position to engage several muscles at once. Plank variations are a fantastic way to build core stability, an essential component for back pain relief and prevention. The core muscles are responsible for stabilizing the spine, so when they are weak, your back can suffer. Performing planks regularly is one of the most effective ways to strengthen these muscles. However, as you build core strength, it's helpful to incorporate different plank variations to target different muscle groups and increase the challenge. Stay tuned to explore several plank variations and how they can help improve core stability and protect your back.

1. The Basic Plank (Forearm Plank)

The basic forearm plank is a great starting point for most people. This exercise works your entire core, including the abdominals, lower back, and hips. It also strengthens the muscles in your shoulders and arms.

To perform a basic forearm plank:

- Start by lying face down on the floor, and then place your forearms on the ground, shoulder-width apart.
- Lift your body up onto your toes and forearms, keeping your body in a straight line from head to heels.
- Engage your core by pulling your belly button toward your spine. Keep your hips level and avoid letting them sag or rise.
- Hold the position for as long as you can, maintaining good form. Start with 20-30 seconds, and work up to longer holds.

This is a great foundation exercise because it activates multiple muscles, helping you build overall stability.

2. Side Plank

The side plank targets the obliques, which are the muscles on the sides of your abdomen. Strengthening your obliques is key to improving side-to-side stability and protecting your back. A strong set of obliques helps prevent twisting motions that can strain your lower back.

To perform a side plank:

- Lie on your side with your legs extended and stacked on top of each other.

- Place your elbow directly under your shoulder, and lift your hips off the ground.
- Keep your body in a straight line from your head to your feet, engaging your core.
- Hold the position for 20-30 seconds on each side.
- For an extra challenge, you can raise your top leg or arm, or perform the side plank with your hand extended rather than your forearm.

This exercise helps you develop strength and stability in the sides of your core, which is crucial for overall spinal health.

3. Plank with Leg Lift

The plank with leg lift is a great variation that adds a challenge to the basic forearm plank by engaging your glutes, lower back, and hip flexors in addition to your core. This helps increase overall core stability and strengthens the muscles that support your lower back.

To perform a plank with leg lift:

- Start in the basic forearm plank position.
- Lift one leg off the ground, keeping it straight and in line with your body.

- Hold the leg up for a few seconds, then lower it back to the ground.
- Repeat on the other side.
- Perform 10-12 reps per side, holding each leg lift for 3-5 seconds.

This variation increases the intensity of the basic plank and challenges your body to maintain stability while lifting one leg at a time.

4. Plank with Arm Lift

Similar to the leg lift variation, the plank with arm lift targets your core, shoulders, and back. Lift one arm to engage your core muscles even more to maintain balance. This variation is particularly helpful for improving upper body strength and enhancing your ability to stabilize your spine.

To perform a plank with arm lift:

- Start in a forearm plank position, keeping your body in a straight line.
- Lift one arm off the ground, reaching it forward or overhead.
- Hold the position for a few seconds, keeping your hips stable.
- Lower the arm back to the floor, and repeat with the other arm.
- Perform 10-12 reps on each side, holding each arm lift for 3-5 seconds.

5. Plank with Knee to Elbow

This variation adds a dynamic element to the plank, incorporating movement that engages your core even more. It helps improve coordination and strengthens the muscles in your abdomen and lower back.

To perform a plank with knee to elbow:

- Start in the forearm plank position.
- Bring your right knee toward your right elbow, then return it to the starting position.
- Repeat with your left knee.
- Perform 10-12 reps on each side.

This variation not only targets the core but also adds a cardio component, making it an excellent full-body exercise.

6. High Plank (Plank on Hands)

The high plank, or plank on hands, is similar to the forearm plank but requires more upper body strength, particularly in your arms, shoulders, and wrists. It challenges your core even further by requiring you to balance on your hands rather than your forearms.

To perform a high plank:

- Start in a push-up position with your hands directly under your shoulders and your feet together.

- Keep your body in a straight line from head to heels.
- Engage your core, avoiding any sagging in your back.
- Hold the position for 20-30 seconds.

This variation is more challenging, requiring a high level of core stability and upper body strength. It's great for building endurance and muscle activation throughout your entire core.

Conclusion

Plank variations are an excellent way to build core strength and stability, both of which are essential for relieving and preventing back pain. As you progress through different variations, your core muscles will become more resilient, reducing the strain on your back and helping you maintain better posture and movement patterns. Start with the basic plank and gradually incorporate more challenging variations to build a strong, stable core that supports your back.

Strategic Suggestions

Incorporating plank variations into your routine will help you develop a strong, stable core that supports your spine and reduces back pain. Progress slowly and maintain good form to build endurance, balance, and strength. A strong core is essential for a healthy back and a pain-free lifestyle.

Bridge Hold: Strengthening the Lower Back

The bridge hold is a powerful exercise that targets the muscles of the lower back, glutes, and hamstrings. This simple yet effective move helps enhance your core stability and supports spinal health. The bridge hold is an excellent exercise for strengthening the muscles that support your lower back. Weakness in these muscles is often a contributing factor to back pain, especially in the lower region of the spine. You'll have to strengthen your glutes, hamstrings, and lower back muscles to create a solid foundation for the spine, helping to reduce discomfort and prevent future injury. The bridge hold not only strengthens the muscles but also improves flexibility, stability, and posture.

Here's how you can safely and effectively perform the bridge hold.

How to Perform the Bridge Hold

Starting Position

Begin by lying on your back on a mat or a comfortable surface, with your knees bent and feet flat on the ground. Your feet should be hip-width apart, and your arms should be resting by your sides with your palms facing down.

Make sure your head, neck, and spine are aligned, and gently engage your core to protect your lower back. Your shoulders should stay relaxed and away from your ears.

Lift the Hips:

- Slowly lift your hips off the floor by pushing through your heels, engaging your glutes and hamstrings. As you lift your hips, your body should form a straight line from your shoulders to your knees.
- Keep your knees from flaring out to the sides, and avoid arching your lower back too much. The goal is to create a neutral spine, which means the natural curve of your lower back is maintained without overextending it.

Hold the Position:

- Once your hips are fully lifted, hold the bridge position for 10-15 seconds. While holding the position, ensure that your glutes and core remain engaged. This helps to strengthen the muscles and protect your lower back.
- Breathe deeply and steadily while maintaining the bridge. Avoid holding your breath, as this can increase tension in your body and hinder your performance.

Lower the Hips:

- Slowly lower your hips back to the starting position, maintaining control over the movement. Avoid letting your lower back sag as you return to the ground.
- Repeat the movement for 10-12 repetitions, or until you feel fatigued. As you build strength, you can gradually increase the duration of the hold or the number of repetitions.

Variations of the Bridge Hold:

As you gain strength and stability, you can incorporate variations of the bridge hold to target different muscles and increase the difficulty level.

1. Single-Leg Bridge Hold:

The single-leg bridge hold is an advanced variation that challenges your balance and engages your core and glute muscles even more. To perform this variation:

- Start in the same position as the standard bridge.
- Lift one leg off the floor while maintaining the bridge with the other leg.

- Hold the bridge position with one leg elevated for 10-15 seconds, then lower your hips and switch legs.
- Perform 5-8 reps on each leg.

This variation requires more strength and stability, particularly in the glutes and core, and helps to enhance the balance between both sides of your body.

2. Bridge Hold with a Squeeze:

Adding a small movement to the bridge hold can make it more effective for strengthening your glutes. For the bridge hold with a squeeze:

- Start in the bridge position, lifting your hips off the ground.
- While holding the bridge, squeeze a small exercise ball or pillow between your knees.

This adds tension to your inner thighs and helps activate the glutes more.

- Hold for 10-15 seconds, then lower your hips.

This variation not only strengthens the glutes but also targets the inner thighs, which play a role in supporting the pelvis and lower back.

3. Bridge Hold with Marching:

For an additional challenge, you can incorporate marching into the bridge hold. This variation helps to further engage your core and hip flexors. To perform it:

- Start in the bridge position.
- Lift one leg off the ground, bringing your knee toward your chest while keeping your hips level.
- Lower that leg and repeat with the other leg.
- Continue alternating for 10-12 reps on each side.

This variation makes your core work harder to maintain stability while your legs move, increasing both the challenge and the benefits.

Why the Bridge Hold Is Effective for Back Health

The bridge hold is especially beneficial for strengthening the muscles in your lower back, hips, and glutes, all of which play a crucial role in supporting your spine. A strong posterior chain (the group of muscles along the back of your body) is essential for maintaining a healthy back and preventing pain.

The lower back is often vulnerable to strain, especially when the muscles that support it are weak. Exercises like the bridge hold, helps to strengthen your glutes and lower back and creates better alignment and stability for your spine. This reduces the risk of pain and injury while improving posture and movement efficiency.

Additionally, the bridge hold can help stretch tight muscles in the lower back and hips, which is important for relieving tension and improving flexibility. Tightness in these areas is a common cause of lower back pain, and regular practice of the bridge hold can help alleviate this discomfort.

Strategic Suggestions

Adding the bridge hold to your routine will help improve core strength, stabilize your lower back, and reduce discomfort. Progress through variations and maintain proper form, so you can build strength and flexibility, helping to prevent and alleviate back pain. Keep consistent, and always focus on controlled movement.

Chapter 4: Lower Body Strength for Spinal Support

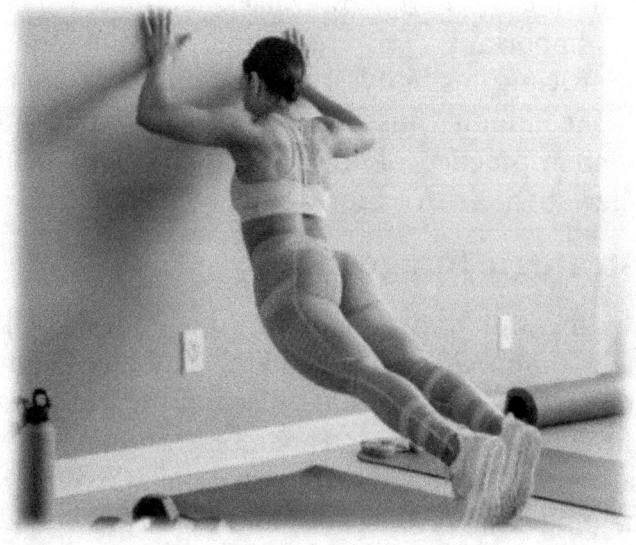

Lower body strength involves the muscles in your legs, hips, and pelvis that help support your spine. Strong lower body muscles are crucial for stabilizing your back, improving posture, and reducing the risk of injury. Strengthening these areas can provide vital support to your spine, enhancing overall back health.

Importance of Lower Body Strength for Back Health

Lower body strength is crucial for overall back health, as it helps support your spine, reduce strain, and prevent injury. Strong legs and hips provide the foundation for proper posture and movement. Your lower body plays a significant role in supporting the health of your spine. It consists of muscles in the legs, hips, and glutes, which work together to stabilize your body and maintain proper posture. When these muscles are weak or imbalanced, they can cause increased stress on your spine, leading to discomfort and pain. Strengthening your lower body is one of the most effective ways to alleviate back pain and prevent future injuries.

The spine itself relies on a network of muscles to stay in alignment and function correctly. If the muscles surrounding your spine aren't strong enough to support it, the spine can become misaligned or subjected to excessive pressure. This misalignment can lead to conditions like herniated discs, muscle strains, and chronic pain. However, strengthening the lower body, particularly the glutes, hamstrings, quadriceps, and hip flexors, helps distribute this pressure more evenly, keeping the spine stable and reducing the risk of injury.

How Lower Body Strength Impacts Your Spine

1. Pelvic Stability

The pelvis serves as the foundation for your spine. When the muscles around the pelvis, such as the glutes and hip flexors, are weak, the pelvis can shift out of alignment. This misalignment can affect the lower back and contribute to pain or discomfort. Strong hip muscles help maintain proper pelvic position, allowing your spine to stay in a neutral, healthy posture.

2. Reduced Stress on the Spine

When you walk, sit, or stand, the muscles in your lower body are responsible for carrying the weight of your upper body. If these muscles are weak, the spine must take on more of the load, which can lead to strain. Build strength in your legs and hips to reduce the strain on your spine, preventing wear and tear on the vertebrae and discs.

3. Better Posture

Poor posture is a common contributor to back pain. Weak lower body muscles can cause an imbalance in your posture, such as slouching or leaning forward, which places excessive pressure on the spine. Strengthening the muscles of your lower body allows for better posture, ensuring that your spine is aligned properly when standing or sitting. A stable and balanced body helps keep your back in a comfortable and pain-free position.

4. Improved Movement Patterns

Proper movement patterns are essential for avoiding strain on your back. When you bend, lift, or move, the muscles of your lower body should be engaged to support your spine. Weak legs or hips can lead to improper movements, such as excessive bending at the lower back or twisting, which increases the risk of injury.

5. Prevention of Back Pain

One of the most significant benefits of lower body strength is the prevention of back pain. Strengthening the lower body helps to prevent the imbalances that often lead to back pain, such as tight hamstrings or weak glutes. A balanced lower body ensures that all the muscles surrounding the spine are working together to keep it healthy. Strong legs, hips, and glutes also improve your ability to recover from minor aches and pains, helping to keep you active and comfortable.

Targeting Key Muscles for Lower Body Strength

To effectively support your back health, it's important to target the key muscle groups in the lower body: the glutes, hamstrings, quadriceps, hip flexors, and calves. Each of these muscle groups plays a vital role in maintaining pelvic stability, proper posture, and overall spinal alignment.

1. Glutes

Strong glutes (the muscles in your buttocks) help stabilize the pelvis and support the lower back. They are essential for movements like standing, walking, and lifting. Weak glutes can lead to an anterior pelvic tilt, which increases pressure on the lower back.

2. Hamstrings

The hamstrings are located at the back of the thighs and help with bending the knees and extending the hips. Tight or weak hamstrings can contribute to back pain by affecting your posture and causing strain on the lower back.

3. Quadriceps

The quadriceps, located at the front of the thighs, help straighten the knee and support the lower body during activities like walking and squatting. Strong quads help balance the load between the front and back of the body, reducing pressure on the spine.

4. Hip Flexors

The hip flexors, located at the front of the hips, are responsible for lifting the legs and bending the hips. Tight hip flexors can lead to an imbalance in posture and contribute to lower back pain, especially if they pull the pelvis out of alignment.

5. Calves

The muscles in your calves help with walking, running, and standing. Strong calves contribute to overall leg strength and stability, reducing the amount of work your lower back has to do.

Exercises for Lower Body Strength

To build strength in your lower body and protect your back, it's essential to incorporate the following exercises into your routine:

1. Squats

Squats are one of the best exercises for building overall lower body strength. They target the quads, glutes, and hamstrings, all of which play a key role in supporting your spine. To perform a squat:

- Stand with your feet shoulder-width apart.
- Bend your knees and lower your hips as if you were sitting in a chair.

- Keep your chest lifted and your back straight as you lower down.
- Return to standing by pushing through your heels.

2. Lunges

Lunges are excellent for targeting the quads and glutes while also improving balance and coordination. To perform a lunge:

- Take a step forward with one foot and bend both knees to lower your hips toward the floor.
- Make sure your front knee stays above your ankle and doesn't extend past your toes.
- Push through your front foot to return to standing, then repeat on the other side.

3. Glute Bridges

As we discussed in earlier sections, glute bridges are excellent for strengthening the glutes and lower back. This exercise helps engage the posterior chain and stabilize the spine.

Conclusion

Lower body strength is a fundamental component of back health. Build strength in your legs, glutes, and hips to provide your spine with the support it needs to stay healthy and pain-free. Incorporating exercises that target these muscle groups into your routine will not only alleviate back pain but also prevent it from recurring. Focus on building strength in your lower body to create a solid foundation for your spine and enjoy better posture, flexibility, and overall back health.

Strategic Suggestions

Incorporating lower body strengthening exercises into your daily routine will not only help alleviate existing back pain but also prevent future discomfort. Focus on exercises like squats, lunges, and glute bridges to build strength and stability in your legs, hips, and glutes. Consistency will help you achieve long-term back health.

Wall Sit: Targeting the Glutes and Quads

The wall sit is a simple yet effective isometric exercise that targets the glutes, quadriceps, and hamstrings, which are all vital for supporting the spine. This exercise helps build endurance and stability in the lower body, providing you with a solid foundation for better posture and a healthier back. The wall sit is a fantastic exercise for strengthening the muscles of your lower body, especially the quadriceps, glutes, and hamstrings.

It's an isometric exercise, meaning you hold a static position to engage the muscles rather than moving through a full range of motion. This makes it a great choice for those looking to build strength without straining the joints or putting unnecessary pressure on the back.

Why the Wall Sit Works

The wall sit primarily targets the quadriceps (the large muscles in the front of your thighs), but it also works your glutes (your butt muscles) and hamstrings (the muscles at the back of your thighs). When you hold a wall sit, these muscles are engaged to keep your body in a stable, seated position, which builds both endurance and strength. Holding this position for an extended period of time helps improve muscle tone and stability, which is especially important for maintaining good posture and protecting your spine.

For back health, the wall sit is particularly beneficial. Strong quads and glutes play a key role in stabilizing the pelvis and spine, reducing the risk of lower back pain and discomfort. Weak quads and glutes can lead to poor posture and misalignment of the pelvis, which puts unnecessary stress on the lower back. The wall sit helps address these muscle imbalances and builds the foundation for proper spinal support.

How to Perform a Wall Sit

1. Find a Wall

Start by standing with your back against a flat wall. Position your feet about hip-width apart and a few inches away from the wall. Ensure that your feet are planted firmly on the ground and facing forward.

2. Slide Down Slowly

Slowly slide your back down the wall, bending your knees until your thighs are parallel to the ground. Make sure your knees are directly above your ankles and not extending past your toes. Keep your back flat against the wall and your core engaged to support your spine. Your knees should form a 90-degree angle, with your thighs parallel to the floor.

3. Hold the Position

Once you've reached the seated position, hold it as long as you can. Keep your feet flat on the floor and your back straight. Focus on engaging your core, quads, glutes, and hamstrings. The longer you hold the position, the more challenging the exercise becomes. Start with shorter durations, such as 20 to 30 seconds, and gradually increase the time as you build strength and endurance.

4. Return to Standing

To finish the exercise, slowly push through your heels to stand back up, using your legs to control the movement. Avoid using your hands or pushing off the wall for assistance. Rest for a few seconds, then repeat the exercise for the desired number of sets.

Key Tips for Success

1. Engage Your Core

To protect your back and improve the effectiveness of the exercise, make sure your core is engaged throughout the wall sit. Imagine pulling your belly button towards your spine to activate your core muscles.

2. Proper Knee Alignment

Avoid letting your knees extend beyond your toes. This can put additional stress on your knees and lower back. Keep your knees stacked directly above your ankles for optimal alignment.

3. Focus on Breathing

While holding the wall sit, it's easy to hold your breath, but it's important to continue breathing steadily. Inhale through your nose and exhale through your mouth to maintain a relaxed state.

4. Challenge Yourself Gradually

Start with short holds, like 20 to 30 seconds, and gradually increase the time as you build strength. Over time, you can work up to holding the position for 1 to 2 minutes or more.

5. Monitor Your Form

Keep your back flat against the wall and avoid slouching. You should feel the muscles in your legs and glutes working, not pain in your lower back. If you experience discomfort in your back, stop and adjust your posture.

Benefits for Back Health

The wall sit strengthens several key muscles that are essential for maintaining a healthy back. Here's how it helps:

1. Pelvic Stability

The wall sit helps stabilize the pelvis by strengthening the glutes, which are responsible for maintaining proper pelvic alignment. When your pelvis is stable, your spine is better supported, reducing the risk of lower back pain.

2. Improved Posture

Strengthening the quads and glutes can help improve your posture, as these muscles support the spine and help maintain an upright, neutral position. A strong foundation in the lower body leads to better spinal alignment and less strain on the back.

3. Reduced Pressure on the Spine

Weak leg muscles force the lower back to take on more weight and pressure, which can lead to discomfort and injury. The wall sit engages and strengthens the muscles of the legs and glutes, reducing the load on the lower back and preventing strain.

4. Endurance and Stability

The wall sit is an isometric exercise, which means it helps build muscular endurance in addition to strength. Endurance is essential for maintaining good posture and reducing fatigue during everyday activities, which can otherwise lead to poor spinal alignment and back pain.

Progressing the Wall Sit

Once you've mastered the basic wall sit, you can progress the exercise in several ways:

1. Increase Duration

Gradually hold the wall sit for longer periods, aiming for 1 to 2 minutes as your endurance improves.

2. Add Resistance

To make the exercise more challenging, you can hold a weight plate or a dumbbell against your chest while performing the wall sit. This additional weight forces the muscles in your lower body to work harder.

3. Single-Leg Wall Sits

For an advanced variation, try lifting one leg off the ground while holding the wall sit. This shifts more of the weight to one side and increases the intensity of the exercise.

4. Wall Sit Marching

Once you're comfortable with holding the wall sit, try lifting one leg at a time in a marching motion while keeping the other leg bent. This adds an element of stability and challenges your core even more.

Strategic Suggestions

The wall sit is a great exercise to strengthen your lower body and support your spine. Target the quads, glutes, and hamstrings to improve posture, reduces strain on the lower back, and enhances endurance. Practice consistently to build a solid foundation for back health and overall stability.

Glute Bridge: Enhancing Hip and Lower Back Strength

The glute bridge is a powerful isometric exercise that targets the glutes, hamstrings, and lower back muscles. When you are able to strengthen these key areas, it helps stabilize the pelvis and lower spine, promoting better posture and alleviating pressure on the lower back. It's a great addition to your back-strengthening routine. The glute bridge is an effective and accessible exercise that can help improve both strength and mobility in the lower back and hips.

This exercise plays a crucial role in supporting the lower spine. A strong, stable pelvis and lower back are essential for maintaining a healthy back and preventing pain.

Why the Glute Bridge Works

The glute bridge is an excellent exercise for strengthening the glutes, hamstrings, and lower back muscles. The glutes are some of the most powerful muscles in the body, and when they are weak, the lower back can become overworked and prone to injury. The glute bridge helps activate these important muscles, improving strength and stability in the hips, pelvis, and lower spine.

In addition to strengthening these key muscles, the glute bridge also improves posture by correcting imbalances. If your glutes are weak, other muscles, like the lower back and hip flexors, can compensate, leading to poor alignment and back discomfort. Strengthen the glutes through the bridge exercise to help restore proper muscle balance, which can alleviate strain on the lower back and prevent pain.

How to Perform a Glute Bridge

1. Start on Your Back

Lie flat on your back on a comfortable surface, like a mat or carpet. Bend your knees and place your feet flat on the floor, about hip-width apart. Your arms should be resting at your sides with palms facing down.

2. Engage Your Core and Glutes

Before you lift your hips, engage your core by pulling your belly button towards your spine. Squeeze your glutes and tighten your abdominal muscles to stabilize your pelvis. This step is crucial to ensure that you are properly activating the right muscles.

3. Lift Your Hips

Push through your heels and raise your hips towards the ceiling, lifting your pelvis off the floor. Your shoulders, hips, and knees should form a straight line at the top of the movement. Be sure to avoid arching your lower back excessively—focus on using your glutes and hamstrings to lift your hips.

4. Hold the Position

Once your hips are raised, hold the position for 2 to 3 seconds, squeezing your glutes at the top. Keep your core engaged and avoid letting your lower back sag. This is the isometric part of the exercise—holding your body in the elevated position will help strengthen the glutes and lower back.

5. Lower Slowly

After holding the bridge position, slowly lower your hips back down to the floor, maintaining control of the movement. Rest for a moment before repeating the exercise.

Key Tips for Success:

1. Mind Your Posture

While performing the glute bridge, avoid arching your lower back or overextending your body. The goal is to use the glutes and hamstrings, not the lower back, to lift the hips. If you feel any strain in your lower back, lower your hips slightly and focus on engaging your glutes more.

2. Feet Placement

Keep your feet flat on the floor, and ensure that your knees are aligned with your hips. Your feet should be positioned about hip-width apart. If your feet are too close to your hips, it may be harder to lift your pelvis; if they are too far, it can place unnecessary strain on your lower back.

3. Slow and Controlled Movements

Perform the exercise slowly and deliberately. The glute bridge is an isometric hold, meaning you should pause at the top of the movement for a few seconds before lowering your hips back down. This helps maximize muscle activation and improves strength.

4. Add Resistance (Optional)

Once you're comfortable with the basic glute bridge, you can increase the intensity by adding resistance. Place a weight plate or a dumbbell on your hips, or use a resistance band looped around your thighs. These modifications will challenge your glutes and hamstrings even more.

5. Breathing

Be mindful of your breathing. Inhale as you prepare to lift your hips, and exhale as you raise your pelvis. Continue breathing steadily throughout the exercise to maintain focus and avoid tension in your body.

Benefits for Back Health

The glute bridge strengthens several key areas that contribute to back health:

1. Strengthens the Glutes and Hamstrings

The glutes and hamstrings play a vital role in stabilizing the pelvis and supporting the spine. When these muscles are weak, the lower back can take on extra load, leading to discomfort and pain. The glute bridge directly targets these muscles, improving their strength and function.

2. Improves Pelvic Stability

A stable pelvis is crucial for maintaining proper alignment in the lower back. The glute bridge strengthens the muscles around the pelvis, including the glutes and hamstrings, which helps keep the pelvis in a neutral position and reduces stress on the spine.

3. Enhances Posture and Alignment

The glute bridge helps improve posture by strengthening the muscles that support the spine and pelvis. When the glutes and hamstrings are strong, they work together to keep the pelvis aligned, which in turn helps prevent lower back pain.

4. Relieves Tight Hip Flexors

Tight hip flexors are a common contributor to lower back pain. The glute bridge helps activate the hip flexors while strengthening the glutes, which can alleviate tightness and improve mobility in the hips and lower back.

Progressing the Glute Bridge

Once you've mastered the basic glute bridge, there are several ways to progress the exercise:

1. Single-Leg Glute Bridge

To make the exercise more challenging, try performing the glute bridge on one leg at a time. This increases the intensity and engages the core more, as you work to stabilize your body with only one leg.

2. Elevated Glute Bridge

Place your feet on a raised surface, such as a bench or step, to perform an elevated glute bridge. This variation increases the range of motion and further activates the glutes and hamstrings.

3. Add Resistance

As with the wall sit, you can add a weight plate or resistance band to increase the challenge.

This will help strengthen the glutes, hamstrings, and lower back even more effectively.

4. Glute Bridge March

Once you've mastered the glute bridge, try alternating leg lifts while holding the bridge position. This adds an element of stability and challenges the core even more.

Strategic Suggestions

The glute bridge is a fantastic exercise for strengthening the glutes, hamstrings, and lower back. Improve muscle balance and pelvic stability to support the spine and alleviate lower back pain. Incorporate this exercise regularly into your routine to enhance overall back health and posture.

Chapter 5: Upper Body and Posture

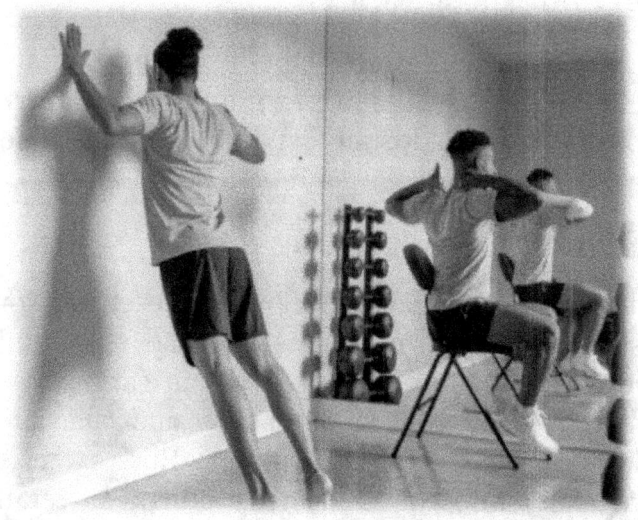

Upper body strength refers to the muscles in your shoulders, arms, and upper back that help support and stabilize your posture. Maintaining strong upper body muscles is essential for preventing back pain, promoting good posture, and ensuring proper alignment of your spine, which reduces strain and supports long-term back health.

The Role of Upper Body Strength in Back Health

Upper body strength plays a crucial role in supporting your back. When the muscles in your upper body are strong, they help maintain proper posture, reduce strain on your lower back, and prevent discomfort. Strong shoulders, arms, and upper back muscles are essential for a healthy spine and pain-free movement.

When we think about back health, we often focus on the lower back and core muscles. However, the upper body also plays an important role in maintaining proper posture, supporting the spine, and preventing back pain. Having strong muscles in the upper body helps create a balanced body that can reduce the strain placed on your lower back.

Upper Body Strength and Posture

Good posture is essential for minimizing back pain. Poor posture—like slouching or rounding your shoulders—puts extra stress on your spine, especially the lower back. When your upper body muscles, including the shoulders, upper back, and chest, are weak, it's harder to maintain proper alignment. This can lead to muscle imbalances, where some muscles become overworked and others become underused. Over time, this imbalance can cause discomfort or pain in your back, neck, and shoulders.

Strong upper body muscles, particularly the ones that stabilize your shoulder blades and support your spine, help keep your posture aligned. These muscles work together to support the spine and maintain an upright position, reducing the load on your lower back. This means that by building strength in the upper body, you can take some of the pressure off your lower back, which can alleviate pain and prevent further injury.

The Importance of Shoulder and Upper Back Strength

The muscles of your upper back, including the traps, rhomboids, and latissimus dorsi, play a critical role in stabilizing the spine and shoulders. These muscles help pull your shoulder blades back and down, which supports the natural curve of your spine. When these muscles are weak, the shoulders tend to round forward, which throws off the alignment of your entire spine.

Strong shoulders also play an important role in maintaining stability and strength when you engage in activities that involve lifting or moving heavy objects. When the shoulders and upper back are weak, these movements can put excessive strain on the lower back, leading to discomfort or injury. Strengthen your upper body to provide your lower back with the support it needs, reducing the risk of strain or injury.

Reducing Strain on the Lower Back

A common cause of lower back pain is poor posture, which can result from weak upper body muscles. When the upper body is not strong enough to hold the spine in proper alignment, the muscles of the lower back have to work harder to compensate. Over time, this added strain can cause muscle fatigue and discomfort in the lower back.

Building strength in your upper body helps to reduce the strain on your lower back muscles. For example, when you strengthen your shoulders and upper back, you help prevent the forward rounding of your shoulders, which can lead to a misalignment of the spine. This alignment helps distribute weight evenly across your body, preventing excess pressure on the lower back.

Upper Body Strength and Spinal Health

The spine is a delicate structure that needs support from all angles. When the muscles in the upper body are weak, the spine is more vulnerable to injury. Strong upper body muscles, particularly those that help stabilize the shoulders and upper back, create a supportive framework that helps keep the spine in its natural alignment.

Muscles like the trapezius, rhomboids, and rotator cuffs work to stabilize the shoulder joints, keeping them in proper alignment with the spine. When these muscles are strong, they help prevent injuries to the shoulder and upper back, which can eventually lead to lower back problems if left unchecked. The muscles that stabilize the shoulders also play a role in reducing neck and upper back strain, both of which can contribute to lower back discomfort.

The Role of the Core in Upper Body Strength

While upper body strength is important, it doesn't work in isolation. The core—comprising the abdominals, lower back, and obliques—works in conjunction with the upper body to maintain stability and prevent strain. If your core is weak, it can put additional stress on your upper body muscles when you move or lift. Strengthening your upper body without addressing the core can create imbalances that may contribute to discomfort or pain.

For example, when lifting or carrying something, the upper body and core muscles must work together to support the spine. If the upper body muscles are weak and the core is not engaged, you may overexert your lower back, leading to pain. A strong core complements upper body strength, allowing for efficient and safe movement patterns that protect the spine and reduce back pain.

How to Build Upper Body Strength for Better Back Health

There are several exercises you can incorporate into your routine to build upper body strength and improve your posture, ultimately benefiting your back health. These exercises should focus on strengthening the muscles of the upper back, shoulders, and arms.

1. Rows

Rows, performed with dumbbells or resistance bands, target the muscles of the upper back, such as the rhomboids and traps. These muscles help pull your shoulders back, improving posture and relieving strain on the lower back.

2. Shoulder Presses

Shoulder presses help strengthen the shoulders and upper arms. Stronger shoulders reduce the tendency to slouch and help maintain proper posture.

3. Lat Pulldowns

Lat pulldowns work the latissimus dorsi muscles, which help stabilize the upper back and support the spine. This exercise strengthens the muscles that help maintain alignment and reduce the risk of back pain.

4. Push-ups

Push-ups target the chest, shoulders, and triceps. They also engage the core, which helps strengthen the upper body and maintain good posture.

5. Reverse Flys

Reverse flys are great for strengthening the muscles of the upper back, particularly the rhomboids and traps. These muscles are essential for stabilizing the shoulder blades and supporting the spine.

6. Chest Openers

Chest openers, such as the chest stretch and doorway stretch, can help counteract the effects of tight chest muscles and forward-rolled shoulders, promoting better posture and reducing strain on the lower back.

Strategic Suggestions

Building upper body strength is essential for supporting your back and maintaining good posture. Strengthen the muscles of your shoulders, upper back, and arms to reduce the strain on your lower back and improve overall spine health. Incorporate upper body exercises to support long-term back health and prevent discomfort.

Wall Pushup: Engaging the Upper Body and Core

Wall pushups are a modified version of the traditional pushup that can help strengthen the upper body and core while being gentler on the back. This exercise targets the chest, shoulders, and triceps, while also engaging the core and stabilizing muscles, promoting better posture and reducing back strain.

Wall pushups are a simple yet effective exercise that can provide numerous benefits for those seeking to improve upper body strength and support back health. Unlike traditional pushups, which require you to be on the floor, wall pushups are performed standing with your hands on a wall or sturdy surface.

How Wall Pushups Benefit Back Health

Wall pushups primarily target the chest, shoulders, and triceps, but they also engage your core, which plays a crucial role in supporting the spine. A strong core helps prevent overcompensation from the back muscles, which can lead to pain and discomfort. When you perform wall pushups correctly, your core activates to stabilize your body as you lower and lift yourself, promoting better posture and reducing strain on the lower back.

In addition to strengthening your upper body, wall pushups also help improve the overall alignment of your body. Poor posture, such as slouching or rounding the shoulders, can put unnecessary pressure on your spine, particularly the lower back. Wall pushups engage the muscles responsible for keeping your shoulders back and your chest open, which encourages better posture and spinal alignment.

Proper Form for Wall Pushups

To get the most out of your wall pushup, it's important to maintain proper form. Here's how to do it correctly:

1. Start Position

Stand facing a wall with your feet about hip-width apart. Place your hands on the wall at shoulder height and slightly wider than shoulder-width apart. Your body should form a straight line from your head to your heels. Keep your feet firmly on the ground and avoid arching your lower back.

2. Engage Your Core

Before you begin the movement, engage your core muscles. This means tightening your abdominal muscles and drawing your navel toward your spine. Engaging your core helps stabilize your body and prevents excessive strain on your lower back.

3. Lowering Your Body

Slowly bend your elbows and lower your chest toward the wall. Keep your body in a straight line as you lower yourself, with your chest coming directly in front of your hands. Make sure your shoulders do not scrunch up toward your ears, and keep your neck in a neutral position.

4. Pushing Back Up

Once your chest is close to the wall, press through your palms to straighten your arms and return to the starting position. Keep your core engaged and avoid letting your lower back sag as you push yourself back up. Focus on using your chest, shoulders, and triceps to power the movement.

5. Breathing

Breathe steadily throughout the exercise. Inhale as you lower yourself toward the wall and exhale as you push back up to the starting position. Proper breathing helps you maintain rhythm and control during the exercise.

Modifying Wall Pushups for Your Needs

If you find wall pushups too challenging or too easy, you can modify the exercise to suit your level of fitness:

To Make it Easier

If you're new to exercise or have limited strength, you can make wall pushups even easier by standing further away from the wall. The further you stand from the wall, the less resistance you'll encounter, which makes the exercise gentler on your muscles and joints.

To Make it Harder

To increase the intensity of the exercise, you can place your feet closer to the wall, making your body more horizontal. You could also perform the pushups with your feet elevated on a step or low platform, increasing the load on your upper body and core. Another option is to slow down the movement, focusing on holding the low point for a few seconds before pushing back up.

Additional Benefits of Wall Pushups

In addition to building upper body strength, wall pushups help improve functional movement patterns that are important for daily activities. Many movements, like pushing, lifting, and carrying, engage the chest, shoulders, and arms. Strengthen these muscles with wall pushups to improve your ability to perform these tasks safely, reducing the risk of injury.

Moreover, wall pushups help engage the core, which is crucial for stabilizing your spine. Strong core muscles allow you to move with more control when you're bending, twisting, or lifting. Engaging your core during wall pushups trains these muscles to work together with your upper body, promoting better movement patterns and reducing strain on your lower back.

Frequency and Progression

To see improvement, aim to include wall pushups in your routine 2-3 times a week. Start with a set of 8-10 repetitions and gradually increase the number as your strength improves. Over time, you can also try performing more sets or progressing to more challenging variations, such as elevated pushups, to continue challenging your muscles and making progress.

Strategic Suggestions

Wall pushups are a great way to build upper body and core strength while reducing strain on your lower back. Maintain proper form and progressively increase the difficulty, so you can improve posture, enhance spinal stability, and help prevent back pain. Incorporate them into your routine for lasting back health benefits.

Shoulder Blade Squeeze: Improving Posture and Stability

The shoulder blade squeeze is a simple yet effective exercise that targets the upper back and shoulders. This exercise helps improve posture, strengthen the muscles responsible for stabilizing the shoulder blades, and promote better spinal alignment. It's a great addition to any routine for enhancing back health and preventing pain.

The shoulder blade squeeze is a straightforward exercise that works wonders for improving posture and strengthening the muscles that support the upper back and neck. These muscles, specifically the rhomboids and trapezius, play a key role in stabilizing the shoulder blades and maintaining a neutral spine. When these muscles are weak, they can contribute to slouching, rounded shoulders, and even back pain.

How the Shoulder Blade Squeeze Benefits Back Health

When you spend a lot of time sitting at a desk, driving, or looking at screens, it's easy for your posture to suffer. Over time, this can lead to a condition called "upper crossed syndrome," which is characterized by rounded shoulders and a forward head posture. The shoulder blade squeeze works to counteract this by strengthening the muscles between your shoulder blades, which helps pull your shoulders back and open up your chest. This helps to reverse the effects of poor posture and reduce the strain on your lower back, neck, and shoulders.

Improving shoulder blade mobility and strength also plays a key role in preventing back pain. Stronger upper back muscles help stabilize the shoulder girdle, reducing the load placed on the spine. A strong upper back allows for better balance and coordination in your movements, which reduces the risk of injury, especially in the lower back.

How to Perform the Shoulder Blade Squeeze

Proper form is essential to get the most benefit from this exercise. Here's how to perform the shoulder blade squeeze correctly:

1. Start Position

Sit or stand up straight with your shoulders relaxed and your arms at your sides. If you're sitting, make sure your feet are flat on the ground and your spine is in a neutral position.

Keep your head aligned with your spine, and engage your core muscles to support your back.

2. Engage the Upper Back

Slowly squeeze your shoulder blades together as though you're trying to pinch a pencil between them. You should feel your upper back muscles working as your shoulder blades move toward each other. Make sure you don't shrug your shoulders up toward your ears.

3. Hold the Squeeze

Hold the squeeze for about 5-10 seconds, focusing on keeping your chest open and your shoulders relaxed. Avoid arching your back as you squeeze; the movement should come from the upper back. Keep your core engaged to help stabilize your spine during the exercise.

4. Release and Repeat

Slowly release the squeeze, allowing your shoulders to return to a neutral position. Take a deep breath and repeat the squeeze. Aim for 10-15 repetitions, depending on your comfort and fitness level. Perform the exercise slowly and with control, focusing on quality over quantity.

Modifications for the Shoulder Blade Squeeze

If you find the standard shoulder blade squeeze too challenging or too easy, you can modify the exercise to suit your needs:

To Make it Easier

If you're new to exercise or experience discomfort in your shoulders, you can try performing the shoulder blade squeeze while lying on your back. This reduces gravity's impact on the muscles and allows you to focus on form and engagement. Lie flat on your back with your arms at your sides and your palms facing upward. Squeeze your shoulder blades together as you would in the seated or standing position.

To Make it Harder

To increase the challenge, you can add resistance to the exercise. One way to do this is by holding a resistance band or light weights in your hands while you perform the shoulder blade squeeze. This adds extra work for the muscles, increasing their strength and endurance. You can also hold the squeeze for longer periods (15-30 seconds) or increase the number of repetitions.

Why Shoulder Blade Squeeze is Crucial for Posture

Good posture isn't just about looking tall and straight; it's about maintaining a balanced and aligned spine. When your shoulder blades are weak and your chest muscles are tight, it becomes harder to maintain proper posture. This misalignment can strain your back, neck, and shoulders, leading to discomfort and pain.

The shoulder blade squeeze targets the muscles responsible for pulling your shoulders back and keeping them in a neutral position. These muscles help counteract the forward hunch caused by prolonged sitting and screen time. Regularly practice shoulder blade squeezes to strengthen these muscles and promote better posture, which in turn reduces stress on the lower back and minimizes the risk of developing back pain.

Additional Benefits of Shoulder Blade Squeezes

Aside from improving posture, the shoulder blade squeeze has other health benefits. It helps enhance shoulder mobility, which is important for preventing stiffness and pain in the shoulder joint. It also helps with scapular stability, which is crucial for proper arm movement during activities like lifting, pushing, or pulling. Strengthening the muscles that support the shoulder blades helps to improve overall shoulder function, making it easier to perform everyday tasks without discomfort.

Incorporating Shoulder Blade Squeezes Into Your Routine

For best results, include shoulder blade squeezes in your daily routine, especially if you spend a lot of time sitting. You can perform them during breaks from work, while watching TV, or as part of your warm-up or cool-down during exercise. It's a low-impact exercise that can be done multiple times a day without causing fatigue or strain.

Strategic Suggestions

Shoulder blade squeezes are a simple yet powerful exercise to strengthen your upper back and improve posture. Incorporate them into your routine, so you can reduce the risk of back pain, improve your spinal alignment, and promote overall stability. Make it a habit for better posture and healthier back muscles.

Chapter 6: Flexibility and Mobility

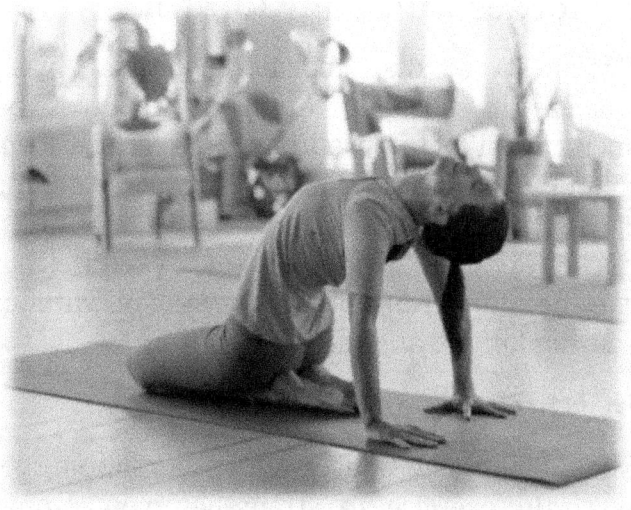

Flexibility refers to the ability of your muscles and joints to move through a full range of motion, while mobility is the ease of movement within that range. Both are crucial for maintaining a healthy back, as they help prevent stiffness, improve posture, and reduce the risk of injury and pain.

The Importance of Flexibility for Back Pain Relief

Flexibility plays a key role in relieving back pain. When your muscles, ligaments, and tendons are flexible, they allow for smooth, natural movements and help reduce tension that can contribute to discomfort. Regular stretching and mobility exercises improve flexibility, promoting healthier posture and a stronger, more balanced back.

Flexibility is often overlooked when managing back pain, but it is one of the most important factors in preventing and relieving discomfort. When we talk about flexibility, we're referring to the ability of your muscles, ligaments, and tendons to stretch and move through a full range of motion. When these structures are tight, they can pull on the spine and other parts of the body, creating imbalances that lead to pain and stiffness. Improving flexibility reduces these tensions, prevents injury, and helps your body move more fluidly.

How Flexibility Affects Your Back Health

Your back is made up of many muscles, ligaments, and joints that need to work together to keep you stable and mobile. If these areas become tight or restricted, they can cause pain and restrict your ability to move freely. For example, tight hamstrings can put more pressure on your lower back, while tight hip flexors can cause you to lean forward in a way that stresses your spine. On the other hand, flexible muscles help maintain proper alignment, reduce tension, and allow for smoother movements that prevent strain.

Flexibility isn't just about being able to touch your toes or do a split. It's about having the right balance of strength and stretch throughout your body, particularly in the muscles surrounding the spine. When your muscles are flexible, they allow for greater mobility in the spine and joints. This makes it easier to maintain good posture, bend, twist, and perform daily activities without triggering pain.

In addition to reducing tension, flexibility also promotes better blood circulation and helps keep muscles relaxed. This means less soreness, fewer spasms, and reduced inflammation around the spine and lower back muscles. Flexibility also supports the nervous system, which can aid in alleviating nerve-related pain, often caused by sciatica or herniated discs.

The Role of Stretching in Flexibility

Stretching is one of the most effective ways to improve flexibility. When you stretch, you are lengthening the muscles, tendons, and ligaments that support your back. This provides relief by releasing tightness and stiffness, which can make movement more fluid and less painful.

There are two main types of stretching: static and dynamic. Static stretching involves holding a stretch for a period of time (typically 15-30 seconds), while dynamic stretching involves moving parts of your body and gradually increasing the range of motion. For back pain relief, a combination of both static and dynamic stretches is beneficial.

Static stretches help lengthen and relax muscles that are tight and tense. Holding these stretches for longer periods allows the muscle fibers to elongate, reducing muscle tightness and promoting flexibility.

Dynamic stretches, on the other hand, help improve mobility by warming up muscles and joints before physical activity. These movements are more controlled, allowing you to move through various positions to increase your range of motion, which reduces stiffness over time.

Key Muscles to Focus on for Back Pain Relief

When it comes to relieving back pain, it's essential to focus on stretching and strengthening key muscles that play a major role in back health. These include the hamstrings, hip flexors, quadriceps, lower back muscles, and the muscles around your shoulders and neck.

1. Hamstrings

Tight hamstrings can pull on the pelvis and cause your lower back to round, creating strain on the spine. Stretching your hamstrings regularly can reduce lower back pain and improve overall flexibility.

2. Hip Flexors

These muscles connect your thighs to your lower back, and they often become tight from prolonged sitting. Tight hip flexors can tilt your pelvis forward, which puts pressure on your lower back. Stretching these muscles helps relieve that pressure and encourages proper spinal alignment.

3. Lower Back Muscles

The muscles along your lower back, including the erector spinae, can become tight from poor posture or overuse. Stretching these muscles can help relieve discomfort and maintain flexibility in the spine.

4. Neck and Shoulders

Tension in your neck and shoulders can radiate down to your back. Stretching your upper body can reduce this tightness and allow for better posture, reducing the likelihood of back pain.

Stretching for Flexibility and Pain Relief

Flexibility exercises should always be done safely to avoid overstretching or straining your muscles. A few tips for stretching safely include:

1. Warm up before stretching

Take 5-10 minutes to do light aerobic activity, like walking or gentle cycling, to warm up your muscles. This makes them more pliable and less prone to injury.

2. Stretch slowly and gently

Stretching too fast or forcing your body into a position can cause muscle strain. Instead, move into each stretch gently and slowly, holding the position without bouncing or jerking.

3. Breathe deeply

Breathing deeply during stretching helps your muscles relax and reduces tension in the body. Inhale as you prepare to stretch, and exhale as you deepen the stretch.

4. Listen to your body

Never push through pain while stretching. If you feel any sharp or intense discomfort, ease off the stretch and try a gentler approach.

Making Flexibility Part of Your Routine

To get the most out of flexibility exercises, aim to incorporate them into your daily routine. Stretching just a few minutes each day can have a huge impact on your back health, reducing pain, preventing stiffness, and improving overall mobility. For those with back pain, it's especially important to target the muscles that directly affect the spine, as well as the muscles that may be compensating for weakness elsewhere in the body.

You can stretch at various times of the day. The key is consistency and gradual improvement, so your body becomes accustomed to the increased range of motion and better flexibility.

Strategic Suggestions

Improving flexibility is essential for managing back pain. Through regular stretching and mobility exercises, you can enhance your posture, prevent stiffness, and relieve discomfort. Make stretching a daily habit for lasting back pain relief, and ensure your muscles stay flexible and strong to support a healthy spine.

Cat-Cow Stretch: Spinal Mobility and Flexibility

The Cat-Cow stretch is a simple yet effective exercise for improving spinal flexibility and mobility. It helps to release tension in the back and neck while encouraging a full range of motion in the spine. This stretch can provide relief from stiffness and promote better posture and alignment.

The Cat-Cow stretch is one of the most accessible and beneficial stretches you can do to improve spinal mobility and relieve back pain. This gentle, flowing movement alternates between arching and rounding your back, which helps to increase the flexibility of your spine and reduce stiffness in your muscles. It's an excellent way to increase spinal mobility, which can help alleviate discomfort, particularly in the lower back. The best part? It's a low-impact stretch that can be done anywhere, and it requires no equipment.

How the Cat-Cow Stretch Works

The Cat-Cow stretch targets the spine and helps to engage the muscles along your back, neck, and torso. As you move through the motion, you alternate between flexion and extension of the spine, which improves the range of motion and relieves tension.

1. Cat Position (Flexion)

In the Cat position, you round your back towards the ceiling, drawing your belly button in and tucking your pelvis under. This position stretches the muscles along the back and helps to release tension in the lower back, especially in the lumbar spine.

2. Cow Position (Extension)

In the Cow position, you arch your back down toward the floor, lifting your head and tailbone toward the sky. This position stretches the front of the body and creates length in the spine, opening up the chest and engaging the muscles along the back.

The combination of both movements—flexion and extension—creates a gentle "massage" for the spine, encouraging blood flow to the muscles and promoting flexibility.

Benefits of the Cat-Cow Stretch for Back Pain

1. Improves Spinal Flexibility and Mobility

The primary benefit of the Cat-Cow stretch is that it increases the flexibility and mobility of the spine. Regular practice of this movement helps your spine move freely and fluidly, reducing stiffness that often leads to back pain.

The alternating motions of rounding and arching encourage flexibility in the thoracic and lumbar spine areas, where tightness can commonly occur.

2. Relieves Tension

This stretch helps to release tension in the muscles of the back, neck, and shoulders. The motion of the Cat-Cow stretch gently massages the spinal muscles, encouraging them to relax and lengthen. This can alleviate discomfort from tight muscles that pull on the spine, contributing to pain and discomfort.

3. Promotes Better Posture

The Cat-Cow stretch helps to realign the spine and improve posture. It involves stretching the back and opening the chest, which is essential for good posture. When you practice this movement regularly, you can reduce the tendency to hunch or slouch, which are common contributors to back pain.

4. Increases Circulation

This dynamic stretch promotes blood flow to the muscles surrounding the spine. Gently move the spine and surrounding muscles, so you can improve circulation and prevent stiffness. Increased blood flow helps deliver nutrients to the muscles and tissues, aiding in healing and reducing inflammation.

5. Prepares the Body for Other Exercises

The Cat-Cow stretch is often used as a warm-up for other stretches or activities that require spinal flexibility. It prepares the back muscles and spine for more challenging movements and helps to prevent injury.

How to Perform the Cat-Cow Stretch

To perform the Cat-Cow stretch correctly, follow these simple steps:

1. Start in a Tabletop Position

Begin by getting on your hands and knees. Your hands should be directly under your shoulders, and your knees should be under your hips. Keep your feet flat on the floor and your back neutral.

2. Cat Pose (Round Your Back)

Inhale deeply, and as you exhale, begin to round your back toward the ceiling. Tuck your chin toward your chest, and pull your belly button toward your spine. Engage your abdominal muscles to help deepen the stretch. This position stretches the muscles along your back and helps to release tension.

3. Cow Pose (Arch Your Back)

Inhale as you slowly begin to reverse the motion. Drop your belly towards the floor, and lift your chest and tailbone towards the ceiling. Look slightly upward, but avoid over-extending your neck. The arch in your back should come from your lower back, not just your upper spine. This position opens the front of the body and lengthens the muscles along your back.

4. Move Between the Two Positions

Flow smoothly between the Cat and Cow positions, inhaling as you arch and exhaling as you round your back. Continue this flow for 5-10 breaths, allowing the stretch to become deeper with each breath. Make sure to keep your movements slow and controlled.

5. Repeat and Hold

As you become more familiar with the movement, you can begin to increase the duration of each hold. Hold each position for 3-5 seconds before transitioning to the other. You can repeat the stretch for 10-15 rounds, depending on how your body feels.

Tips for Safe and Effective Practice

1. Focus on Breath

Make sure to synchronize your breath with the movement. Inhale as you arch your back (Cow pose) and exhale as you round your back (Cat pose). Focusing on your breath helps to relax your muscles and deepen the stretch.

2. Move Slowly

Avoid rushing through the movements. The Cat-Cow stretch is most effective when done slowly and deliberately. Allow your body to move freely and fluidly between the two positions, without forcing the motion.

3. Listen to Your Body

If you feel any discomfort or pain, ease off the stretch or adjust your positioning. Always work within your own range of motion and avoid pushing your body too far.

4. Add Variations

Once you become comfortable with the standard Cat-Cow stretch, you can explore variations, such as adding gentle side-to-side movements or incorporating small circles with your hips to further increase mobility.

Making the Cat-Cow Stretch Part of Your Routine

To maximize the benefits of the Cat-Cow stretch, try to incorporate it into your daily routine. It's a simple, quick stretch that can be done in the morning to wake up the spine or before bed to release tension from the day. You can also use it as a warm-up before more intense exercises or to relieve back pain throughout the day.

Strategic Suggestions

The Cat-Cow stretch is an excellent way to improve spinal mobility and relieve back pain. Practicing it regularly can help increase flexibility, reduce tension, and improve posture. Add this simple exercise to your daily routine to promote a healthier back and better overall movement throughout your day.

Seated Forward Fold: Stretches for Hamstrings and Lower Back

The Seated Forward Fold is a gentle stretch that targets the hamstrings and lower back. This simple yet effective stretch helps to release tension, improve flexibility, and alleviate discomfort in the back. The Seated Forward Fold (also known as Paschimottanasana in yoga) is a deep stretch that focuses on the hamstrings, lower back, and spine. It's one of the most effective exercises for improving flexibility in the lower body and promoting relaxation throughout the entire back.

No matter if you're dealing with tight hamstrings, lower back pain, or just looking to increase flexibility, the Seated Forward Fold is a wonderful addition to your routine. The beauty of this stretch lies in its simplicity and accessibility. You don't need any equipment or a lot of space to do it, and it can be performed at any time during the day.

How the Seated Forward Fold Helps

The Seated Forward Fold is a powerful stretch for several reasons:

1. Targets the Hamstrings

Tight hamstrings are a common contributor to lower back pain. When the muscles in the back of your legs are tight, they pull on the pelvis and cause discomfort in the lower back. The Seated Forward Fold lengthens these muscles, helping to reduce tension and strain on the lower back.

2. Stretches the Spine

As you fold forward, the stretch lengthens the spine, improving its flexibility. The gentle stretching motion helps to release tension in the muscles surrounding the spine, particularly the lower back and lumbar area. This can lead to reduced stiffness, increased range of motion, and relief from pain.

3. Promotes Relaxation

This stretch is not only effective for improving flexibility but also for calming the body and mind. The Seated Forward Fold helps to promote relaxation. This is especially beneficial if you're experiencing stress-related tension in your lower back.

4. Improves Posture

By stretching both the hamstrings and the lower back, the Seated Forward Fold helps to create better alignment in the spine. Improved flexibility in these areas can lead to better posture overall, reducing the likelihood of developing poor posture that leads to back pain.

How to Perform the Seated Forward Fold

Here's a step-by-step guide to performing the Seated Forward Fold correctly:

1. Start Seated with Legs Extended

Begin by sitting on the floor with your legs extended straight in front of you. Keep your feet flexed, with your toes pointing upward, and ensure your knees are straight. Sit up tall with a long spine and your shoulders relaxed.

2. Engage Your Core

Before you begin folding forward, engage your core muscles. Draw your belly button gently towards your spine to support your lower back as you begin the fold. This helps protect your spine and allows for a deeper stretch without straining.

3. Inhale and Lengthen the Spine

Take a deep breath in and, as you do, lengthen your spine. Imagine reaching the crown of your head toward the ceiling, which helps to elongate your torso and create space in your spine. It's important to maintain this length throughout the stretch to avoid rounding your back prematurely.

4. Exhale and Fold Forward

As you exhale, gently fold forward at your hips, not your lower back. Imagine hinging at the waist, leading with your chest and stomach rather than your head. Avoid rounding your back excessively—keep it long and straight as you reach for your feet, ankles, or shins, depending on your flexibility.

5. Hold the Stretch

Once you've reached a comfortable position, hold the stretch for 15-30 seconds, breathing deeply and allowing your body to relax into the fold. If you can't reach your feet right away, that's okay! Just place your hands on your shins, ankles, or the floor beside your legs, and focus on lengthening your spine with each breath.

6. Deep Breathing

Throughout the stretch, remember to focus on deep, even breathing. As you breathe in, try to lengthen your spine even more. As you breathe out, deepen the fold slightly, but only to a point where it feels comfortable—never force the stretch.

7. Release the Stretch

To come out of the stretch, slowly and gently roll your spine back up, stacking each vertebra one at a time, until you are sitting upright again. Take a moment to sit tall, feeling the stretch in your hamstrings and lower back. Repeat the stretch 2-3 times for maximum benefit.

Tips for Safe and Effective Practice

1. Don't Force the Stretch

It's important to avoid forcing yourself into a deeper fold if your body isn't ready. Stretching should never feel painful. Always work within your own range of motion and listen to your body.

2. Use a Prop

If you can't reach your feet or if your hamstrings are very tight, use a yoga strap or belt around your feet to help deepen the stretch without overextending your reach. You can also place a cushion or bolster under your knees for added comfort.

3. Keep a Long Spine

One of the most common mistakes in the Seated Forward Fold is rounding the back too much. Instead of folding from your lower back, focus on hinging at the hips and keeping your spine long. This will ensure you're targeting the correct muscles and avoiding strain.

4. Practice Consistency

Like any flexibility exercise, the Seated Forward Fold requires consistent practice. Over time, you'll notice your hamstrings and lower back becoming more flexible, leading to improved posture and decreased discomfort.

Benefits Beyond the Lower Back

The Seated Forward Fold doesn't only target the lower back and hamstrings; it also has benefits for other parts of the body, including the calves and even the upper body. This stretch helps to release tension throughout the body. As you deepen the stretch with each breath, your body will begin to relax, which can help to reduce overall stress levels. It's a great stretch to do during breaks from sitting or before bed to promote relaxation.

Strategic Suggestions

The Seated Forward Fold is an excellent way to stretch your hamstrings and lower back. Incorporate this stretch into your routine to improve flexibility, reduce back pain, and create better posture. Practice it consistently to experience long-term benefits for your back health and overall well-being.

Chapter 7: Functional Movements and Back Health

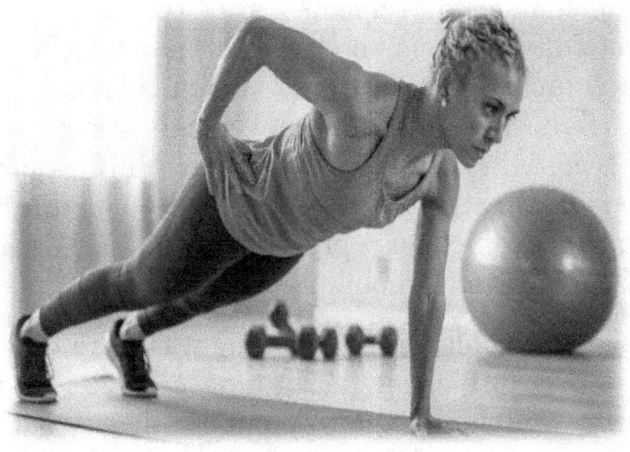

Functional movements are everyday activities that require strength, stability, and coordination, such as bending, lifting, and twisting. They are crucial for back health because they train your body to move efficiently and safely, reducing the risk of strain or injury while improving overall flexibility and muscle balance for long-term back support.

The Connection Between Functional Movements and Back Health

Functional movements are the everyday motions that your body performs naturally to accomplish routine tasks. When it comes to back health, functional movements are crucial because they mimic how you move during daily activities. Strengthening the body with these movements helps prevent back pain and improve overall mobility.

When it comes to maintaining a healthy back, it's not just about performing exercises in a gym or following a workout routine. What's equally important is how you move during daily life. Functional movements are the foundation of this. They are the motions that help us perform essential tasks, such as bending, lifting, walking, and twisting. These movements are natural, often subconscious, and they closely mimic what our bodies are designed to do in the real world.

For example, think about the simple act of picking something up from the floor. It seems like an easy task, but it requires the coordination of your back, core, and legs. If you haven't trained your body to move correctly, this seemingly harmless task could result in strain and injury. This is where functional movements come into play. When your body is prepared for the tasks it performs daily, you're less likely to experience pain or discomfort.

Functional movements play a significant role in preventing and managing back pain. These movements focus on activating the muscles and joints you rely on the most. They can help improve your posture, enhance stability, and ensure you move in a way that protects your spine. Having a solid foundation in functional movement patterns helps you avoid bad habits, like slouching, that contribute to back pain.

One of the main reasons functional movements are effective for back health is because they engage multiple muscle groups at once. This coordinated effort strengthens not just the back but also the core, legs, and arms. A well-developed core, for example, is key for protecting your spine and reducing strain on your lower back. Think of your core as the body's natural support system – a strong core is like having a built-in brace for your spine.

Functional exercises can also improve flexibility and mobility. When you incorporate functional movements into your routine, you improve the range of motion in your muscles and joints. This increased mobility allows for better movement patterns in daily tasks, reducing stiffness and discomfort, especially in the lower back and hips.

Additionally, functional movements train your body to be more stable. Stability is essential for maintaining proper posture and avoiding excessive pressure on your spine. Many back problems arise when the body's stabilizing muscles are weak or inactive. Functional movements help activate these stabilizing muscles, so they can properly support your spine during activities that involve bending, lifting, or twisting.

So how do you begin incorporating functional movements into your daily life to improve your back health? One of the simplest ways to start is by practicing safe movement techniques. This can include learning how to squat properly, how to lift an object with your legs instead of your back, or how to engage your core when you stand up or sit down.

It's important to recognize that the benefits of functional movements extend beyond preventing back pain. They contribute to overall well-being. As you strengthen your muscles and improve your movement patterns, you'll notice increased energy, reduced fatigue, and an improved quality of life. Functional movements keep the body agile and capable of handling whatever daily tasks you face.

Incorporate functional movements into your exercise routine and daily habits to set yourself up for a stronger, healthier back. You're also reducing your chances of injury, ensuring that your spine remains well-supported throughout your lifetime.

Strategic Suggestions

To improve your back health and prevent pain, make functional movements a regular part of your routine. Begin by practicing proper lifting techniques and engaging your core when moving. Over time, incorporate more exercises that mimic daily motions to strengthen your back, core, and legs for lasting support.

Standing Deadlift Hold: Strength and Balance

The standing deadlift hold is a powerful isometric exercise that focuses on strengthening your core, legs, and back while improving balance and stability. This exercise is simple to perform and can significantly contribute to better posture and reduced back pain when practiced regularly. The standing deadlift hold is an isometric exercise, meaning it involves holding a position rather than performing dynamic movements. This exercise primarily targets the muscles of the posterior chain—the back, glutes, hamstrings, and core—making it particularly effective for improving posture and reducing lower back pain.

When done correctly, the standing deadlift hold can also enhance your balance and stability, both of which are crucial for preventing injury during everyday activities.

Here's how to perform the standing deadlift hold:

1. Position Your Feet and Hips

Begin by standing tall with your feet hip-width apart. Keep a slight bend in your knees to avoid locking them. Your feet should be flat on the ground, with your toes pointing straight ahead.

2. Engage Your Core

Before starting the movement, tighten your core muscles. Imagine pulling your belly button toward your spine to create a stable base for your body. Engaging your core is essential to protect your lower back throughout the exercise.

3. Hinge at the Hips

To begin the movement, push your hips back as if you were reaching to pick something up off the floor. This is a hip-hinge movement, not a squat. Your knees will bend slightly, but your hips will do the majority of the work. Keep your back straight and your chest lifted throughout.

4. Hold the Position

As you hinge your hips back, stop when your torso is about parallel to the ground, or as far as your mobility allows without rounding your back. Your arms should hang naturally at your sides. Hold this position for 20-30 seconds, making sure to maintain good form throughout.

5. Return to Standing

After holding the position, slowly and with control, return to a standing position by pushing through your heels and driving your hips forward. Do not rush this movement; take your time to avoid straining your back.

The key to this exercise is maintaining proper posture and alignment while holding the position. Keeping your spine neutral, your core engaged, and your knees slightly bent ensures that the exercise targets the right muscle groups and reduces the risk of injury. Additionally, you should never allow your back to round during the hold. If you find yourself unable to maintain a neutral spine, reduce the depth of your hinge until you can hold proper form.

Benefits for Back Health

The standing deadlift hold offers several important benefits for your back health:

1. Strengthens the Posterior Chain

The muscles of the posterior chain, including the lower back, glutes, and hamstrings, are essential for maintaining good posture and proper alignment. Strengthening these muscles can help alleviate pressure on your spine and reduce the risk of back pain.

2. Improves Balance and Stability

This exercise challenges your balance by requiring you to hold a static position while engaging multiple muscle groups. This improves your ability to maintain stability in other activities, such as walking, standing, or lifting objects.

3. Enhances Core Engagement

Your core plays a crucial role in supporting your back and maintaining good posture. The standing deadlift hold requires you to engage your core muscles, helping to improve core strength and reduce the strain on your lower back.

4. Increases Flexibility in the Hamstrings

Holding the hip-hinge position in the deadlift stretch helps to lengthen and stretch the hamstrings. Tight hamstrings are often associated with back pain, so incorporating this movement can help improve flexibility and reduce discomfort.

5. Promotes Better Posture

Regularly practicing the standing deadlift hold can help reinforce proper posture by strengthening the muscles responsible for keeping your spine in alignment. Better posture leads to less strain on your back, improving both comfort and mobility.

6. Reinforces Hip-Hinge Movement

The standing deadlift hold teaches proper hip-hinge mechanics, which is an essential movement pattern for daily activities like bending down, picking up objects, or standing up from a seated position. Mastering the hip hinge helps prevent poor posture and reduces the likelihood of injury.

Strategic Suggestions

To make the most of the standing deadlift hold, focus on keeping your form correct throughout the exercise. Gradually increase the time you hold the position as your strength and balance improve. Consistency with this exercise will help you build a strong, stable foundation for a healthy back and improve your overall movement patterns.

BirdDog Hold: Core and Back Integration

The BirdDog hold is an isometric exercise that engages both your core and back muscles, making it an excellent movement for improving stability and strength. This exercise plays a crucial role in alleviating back pain and preventing further injury. The BirdDog hold is an excellent exercise for enhancing both core strength and spinal stability. This move involves holding a balanced position where you extend opposite arm and leg, working together to engage your core, back, and hips. It is a dynamic exercise in that it challenges you to maintain stability while stretching and strengthening your back muscles.

Here's how to perform the BirdDog hold:

1. Get Into Starting Position

Begin on all fours with your hands under your shoulders and knees under your hips. Ensure your wrists are directly beneath your shoulders and your knees are directly beneath your hips. This is a neutral, balanced position that allows you to move freely without straining your joints.

2. Engage Your Core

Before moving your arms or legs, tighten your core muscles. Imagine pulling your belly button toward your spine to create a stable base. Engaging your core is crucial for preventing any lower back strain during the movement.

3. Extend Opposite Arm and Leg

Slowly extend your right arm forward while simultaneously extending your left leg straight back. Keep your arm and leg level with your body, as if you were reaching forward and backward in opposite directions. Avoid arching your back or allowing your hips to rotate. Both should remain square to the floor.

4. Hold the Position

Once your arm and leg are fully extended, hold the position for 20-30 seconds. Keep your head in a neutral position, looking down at the floor, and ensure your neck remains aligned with your spine. During the hold, focus on maintaining balance and stability through your core and back muscles.

5. Return to Starting Position

Slowly bring your arm and leg back to the starting position. Take a moment to reset and engage your core before performing the other side. Repeat the movement by extending your left arm and right leg, holding the position for the same amount of time.

The BirdDog hold requires you to focus on keeping your back and hips stable while extending your limbs. It's easy to let your lower back dip or your hips rotate, but maintaining a neutral spine is key to avoiding injury and achieving the best results.

Benefits for Back Health

The BirdDog hold provides numerous benefits for your back health, particularly in terms of strengthening and stabilizing your core and lower back. Here are the key benefits:

1. Core Stability

The primary benefit of the BirdDog hold is its ability to strengthen your core muscles, including your abdominals, obliques, and lower back muscles. A strong core is vital for maintaining good posture and supporting your spine, which helps to prevent or alleviate back pain.

2. Improved Balance

The BirdDog hold challenges your balance by requiring you to maintain a stable position while extending opposite limbs. This improves proprioception (your sense of body position in space), which can help you perform everyday activities with better posture and fewer chances of injury.

3. Back Muscle Engagement

The exercise specifically targets the muscles in your lower back, glutes, and hips. Strengthening these muscles helps relieve pressure from your spine and reduces the risk of injury.

4. Posture Correction

Consistent practice of the BirdDog hold encourages better posture by reinforcing the alignment of the spine and pelvis. Over time, this can reduce slouching or poor posture habits that contribute to back pain.

5. Lower Back Pain Relief

The BirdDog hold strengthens and stabilizes the muscles around your lower back, reducing strain and pressure. This exercise engages your core muscles, helping to improve spinal alignment, which can alleviate lower back pain.

6. Prevents Hip Imbalances

The BirdDog hold helps address any imbalances in your hips. Since one leg is extended while the opposite arm is extended, both sides of the body are engaged, leading to more balanced strength in the hip and core muscles.

7. Enhanced Coordination

The BirdDog hold requires coordination between your arms, legs, and core muscles. This integration helps improve overall functional movement, making daily activities like lifting, bending, or walking feel easier and more controlled.

8. Improved Spinal Health

The BirdDog hold promotes spinal stability by strengthening the muscles that support your spine. A strong, well-supported spine reduces the likelihood of experiencing back pain and improves overall mobility.

Strategic Suggestions

To get the most out of the BirdDog hold, focus on keeping your body in a straight line, from your head down to your extended foot. Gradually increase the duration of each hold as your strength and stability improve. If you're new to this exercise, start with short holds and focus on form. As you become more comfortable, aim for longer durations to enhance your core and back health. Consistent practice will help you develop the stability needed for a pain-free, active lifestyle.

Chapter 8: Advanced Isometric Exercises for Back Strength

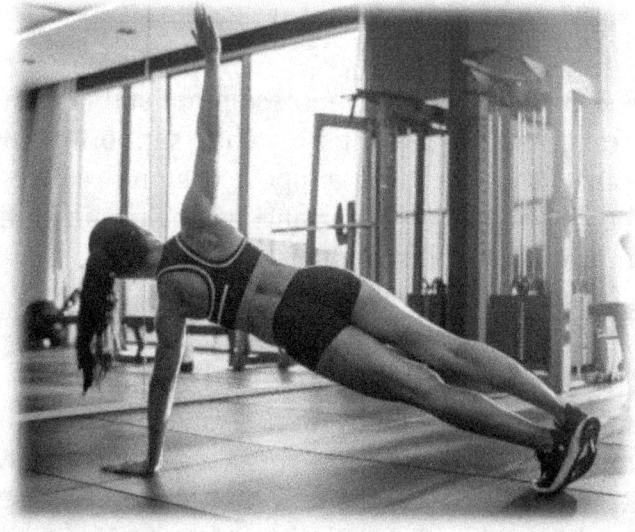

Advanced isometric exercises involve holding more challenging positions that require increased strength and endurance to engage deeper muscle groups. These exercises are vital for building back strength, improving stability, and preventing injury. Incorporating them into your routine can take your back health to the next level, providing long-term support and resilience.

Advanced Plank Variations for Maximum Core Stability

The plank is one of the most effective exercises for building core strength. When you hold your body in a straight line while balancing on your forearms or hands, you engage your abdominal muscles, back, and even your glutes. But if you're already comfortable with the standard plank, advancing it can help build even greater strength and stability in your core, which is essential for a healthy back. A weak core can lead to poor posture and imbalances, putting undue stress on the spine. Plank variations are a great way to increase core strength and maximize your body's ability to stabilize your back.

Here are a few advanced plank variations that can take your core training to the next level. As you progress, your body will become more adept at handling the strain, and your muscles will grow stronger.

1. Plank with Leg Lifts

One of the simplest ways to make the plank more challenging is by adding leg lifts. Start in a regular forearm plank position, ensuring your body forms a straight line from your head to your heels. Keeping your hips stable, lift one leg off the floor as high as you can while maintaining your body's alignment. Hold for a few seconds, then lower the leg and repeat with the other side. This move engages not only your abs but also your glutes and lower back muscles, enhancing both core and spinal stability.

Tip: Keep your hips level throughout the exercise. Avoid letting your back sag or your hips rise too high. This ensures you're working your core effectively.

2. Side Plank with Leg Raise

The side plank is a great variation that focuses more on your obliques, the muscles along the sides of your torso. To do this, lie on your side with your forearm directly under your shoulder, your legs stacked on top of each other, and your body in a straight line. Once you lift your hips off the floor, hold this position. For added challenge, lift your top leg up toward the ceiling. This variation targets your core muscles even more and also works your hips, glutes, and shoulders.

Tip: Keep your shoulder, hip, and ankle in a straight line. Focus on lifting your leg with control, not just for height but also to engage your core.

3. Plank with Arm Reaches

Adding arm movements to the plank increases the challenge by requiring more balance and stability. Start in a forearm plank position and reach one arm forward, extending it straight in front of you. Hold this position for a few seconds, then lower the arm and repeat with the other arm. This variation forces your core to engage even more to maintain your stability while you lift your arm off the ground. The additional arm movement simulates more real-world conditions and makes the exercise more dynamic.

Tip: Keep your hips and shoulders square to the floor as you reach your arm out. Avoid twisting or rotating your body.

4. Plank to Push-Up

If you want to really challenge your upper body while continuing to work your core, the plank to push-up variation is an excellent choice. Start in a forearm plank position, then push up onto your hands one arm at a time, until you're in a full plank position. From here, lower back down onto your forearms, again one arm at a time. This movement requires a high level of coordination, upper body strength, and core stability. It also engages your chest, shoulders, and triceps while continuing to target your abdominals and back.

Tip: When transitioning between forearm and hand positions, try to keep your movements smooth and controlled. Do not rush through the exercise.

5. Plank with Knee to Elbow

This variation adds more dynamic movement to your standard plank. Start in a regular plank position, either on your hands or forearms, and bring one knee toward the opposite elbow while keeping your body straight. As you bring your knee in, engage your core muscles to maintain stability. Alternate sides and repeat. This movement intensifies the challenge by incorporating your obliques and hip flexors while continuing to activate your abs and lower back muscles.

Tip: Keep your back flat as you bring your knee in. Try to avoid letting your hips dip or lift as you move.

Strategic Suggestions

When practicing these advanced plank variations, remember that form is key to avoiding injury and maximizing benefits. Begin with simpler variations, then gradually move to more challenging ones as your strength increases. Regular practice will build your core stability, which can significantly improve your posture, relieve back pain, and enhance your overall fitness. Always listen to your body and ensure you're engaging the correct muscles for the best results. Consider pairing these plank variations with other back-strengthening exercises for a comprehensive workout that promotes back health and pain relief.

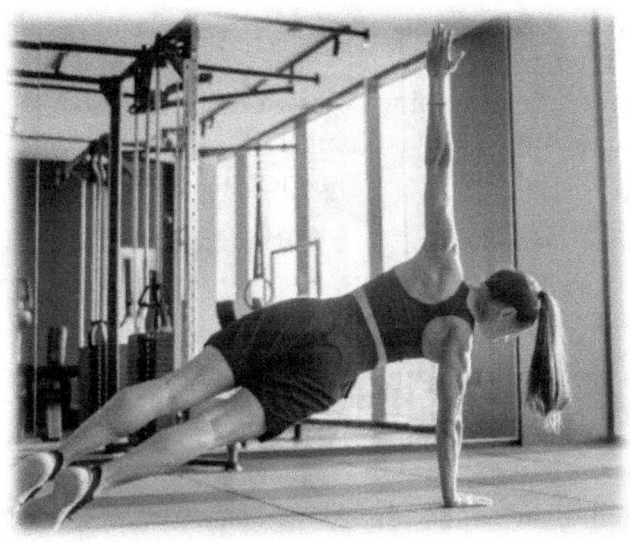

Wall Squat Hold: Increasing Endurance and Strength

The wall squat hold is a simple but powerful exercise that targets your lower body, specifically the quads, hamstrings, and glutes. It is an excellent way to build endurance and strength in your legs while also helping to support your spine. When done correctly, wall squat holds can enhance overall stability and contribute to long-term back health.

Wall squats are a great isometric exercise because they allow you to work your leg muscles while keeping your back in a supported position. Unlike many other exercises, the wall squat hold doesn't require complex movements, making it a great option for people of all fitness levels. It's especially helpful for individuals with back pain since it works to strengthen the muscles that support the spine.

Here's how to perform the wall squat hold:

1. Position Yourself Against the Wall

To start, stand with your back against a wall, your feet about 12-18 inches in front of you. Your feet should be shoulder-width apart, and your toes should point forward. Slowly slide your back down the wall while keeping your body in a straight line, bending your knees as if you're sitting in a chair.

Tip: Ensure your knees are directly above your ankles, and avoid letting them extend past your toes. Keep your chest lifted, and don't round your back. It's important to keep your back in contact with the wall at all times to avoid straining your lower back.

2. Hold the Position

Once your thighs are parallel to the ground, or slightly lower if you're able, hold the position. Your legs should form a 90-degree angle at the knees. Engage your core to help keep your back stable and reduce pressure on your spine. Keep your weight evenly distributed between your heels and the balls of your feet. Hold the position for 30 seconds to a minute, depending on your fitness level.

Tip: Keep your abs tight and avoid leaning forward or backward. Focus on maintaining a flat back against the wall throughout the exercise.

3. Breathing and Core Engagement

While holding the wall squat position, it's essential to focus on controlled breathing. Exhale as you sink deeper into the squat and inhale as you hold steady. Engaging your core during the hold is critical for ensuring that you don't place excessive pressure on your spine. It will also help protect your lower back from potential strain.

Progression and Modification

The wall squat hold can be progressed by increasing the hold time or by adding variations. Once you've mastered the basic squat hold, you can challenge yourself by:

1. Adding a leg lift

Lift one leg slightly off the ground while holding the squat position. This will engage your core even more and challenge your balance.

2. Using a resistance band

Place a resistance band around your thighs just above your knees. As you squat down, press your knees outward against the resistance band to increase the challenge to your outer thighs and hips.

3. Holding the squat longer

Gradually increase the amount of time you hold the squat to build more endurance.

Tip: Start with short holds and gradually increase the time as your muscles become more accustomed to the challenge. Make sure you don't compromise form for duration. Proper form is essential for maximizing the benefits and preventing injury.

Benefits for Back Health

While the wall squat primarily targets the lower body, its benefits extend to your back health as well. Stronger quads, hamstrings, and glutes provide better support for your spine. These muscles help stabilize the pelvis and prevent unnecessary strain on the lower back during daily activities. Incorporate wall squats into your routine to train your lower body to take some of the load off your spine, which can alleviate back pain and improve overall posture.

Strategic Suggestions

The wall squat hold is a highly effective exercise for building lower body strength and improving back health. As you progress, aim to increase your hold time and add variations to make the exercise more challenging. It's important to stay mindful of your form to avoid any strain on your back. Integrate the wall squat hold into your routine alongside other exercises targeting core and back strength for a balanced approach to back health. Always listen to your body and adjust the intensity of the exercise as needed.

Superman Hold: Strengthening the Entire Back

The Superman hold is a powerful isometric exercise that targets the entire back, including the lower back, upper back, glutes, and shoulders. It's an excellent way to build strength and stability throughout your spine, helping to alleviate back pain and improve posture. The Superman hold is named after the superhero pose, as it involves lying face down and lifting your arms and legs off the ground, mimicking the flying position of Superman.

This exercise works a variety of muscle groups simultaneously, making it a great addition to any fitness program, especially if you're looking to relieve back pain or prevent future injuries.

Here's how to perform the Superman hold:

1. Start in the Right Position

Begin by lying face down on a mat or a comfortable surface with your arms extended in front of you and your legs straight. Your forehead should be resting lightly on the floor, and your body should be in a neutral, straight line. It's important to keep your head, neck, and spine aligned to avoid straining your neck during the exercise.

Tip: Ensure that your body is fully extended, with your arms and legs reaching out as far as they comfortably can. This will help activate all the muscles you intend to target in the back.

2. Lift Your Arms and Legs

Slowly raise your arms and legs off the ground simultaneously, focusing on lifting your chest, thighs, and feet as high as possible without straining your lower back. Your goal is to keep your body in a gentle "arched" position while maintaining full engagement of your core and back muscles.

Tip: Keep your arms extended, palms facing down, and legs straight. As you lift, think about pulling your arms and legs away from each other to maximize muscle engagement.

3. Engage Your Core and Back Muscles

While holding this position, engage your core to support your spine. Contract your glutes, lower back muscles, and upper back muscles to maintain the lift. Keep your chest and thighs elevated, and avoid letting your arms and legs drop. Hold the position for 20-30 seconds to start, then gradually increase your hold time as you get stronger.

Tip: Focus on squeezing your glutes and lower back muscles to maintain the lifted position.

4. Breathing

Breathing while holding the Superman pose is crucial for maintaining form and preventing unnecessary tension in your muscles. Take slow, controlled breaths as you hold the position. Inhale deeply as you lift your arms and legs, then exhale gently as you hold the pose. Try not to hold your breath, as it could cause unnecessary strain on your body.

Progression and Modification

As you get stronger, you can increase the difficulty of the Superman hold by:

1. Increasing the hold time

Start with 20-30 seconds and gradually increase the duration to 1-2 minutes as your strength and endurance improve.

2. Adding variations

For a greater challenge, you can alternate lifting each arm and leg. Lift one arm and the opposite leg simultaneously, hold for a few seconds, and then alternate. This variation adds a balance component that engages the core even more.

3. Weighted variation

For advanced practitioners, you can add ankle weights or a light resistance band to further challenge your back muscles.

Tip: Focus on quality over quantity when performing the Superman hold. It's better to hold the position for a shorter period with proper form than to strain yourself by holding too long with poor technique.

Benefits for Back Health

The Superman hold is highly effective for strengthening the muscles of the back, which are essential for supporting the spine and maintaining proper posture. Engage your glutes, lower back, and upper back muscles to improve stability throughout the entire back. This can help alleviate back pain, prevent future injuries, and improve your ability to perform daily tasks with ease. The exercise also helps balance muscle imbalances that may be contributing to poor posture and back discomfort.

The Superman hold also targets the muscles that support your spine, helping to reduce the risk of slouching and improper posture. Over time, strengthening these muscles leads to improved posture, less back pain, and a more aligned spine.

Strategic Suggestions

The Superman hold is a fantastic exercise for targeting the muscles of your back and core. Gradually increase your hold time and incorporating variations, so you can continue to challenge yourself and improve your back strength. Remember to focus on your form and engage the right muscles to avoid any strain. As you strengthen your back, you'll notice improved posture, less pain, and greater overall stability. Incorporate the Superman hold into your routine for a stronger, more resilient back, and be mindful of progressing at your own pace to achieve lasting results.

Chapter 9: Nutrition and Hydration for Back Health

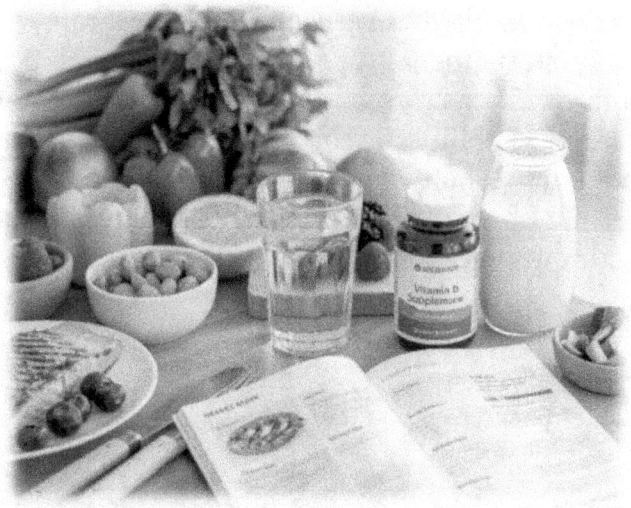

Nutrition refers to the intake of essential vitamins, minerals, and nutrients that support overall health, while hydration is the process of maintaining adequate fluid levels in the body. Both are crucial for back health, as proper nutrition and hydration reduce inflammation, promote tissue repair, and ensure muscles and joints function optimally.

Antiinflammatory Foods for Pain Relief

Back pain can be incredibly debilitating, and while exercise plays a vital role in strengthening muscles, the food you eat can also significantly impact your recovery. Consuming anti-inflammatory foods can help reduce pain, swelling, and stiffness in your back. These foods can not only provide relief but also promote overall health and wellbeing.

The link between nutrition and back pain is stronger than many realize. When your body experiences inflammation, it can lead to pain and discomfort in various parts, including your back. Include anti-inflammatory foods in your diet, so you can help reduce this inflammation, providing relief to your back muscles and joints.

The body's inflammatory response is natural; it's part of how your immune system reacts to injury or infection. However, chronic inflammation, especially in the muscles and tissues around the spine, can cause long-term pain and discomfort. A diet rich in anti-inflammatory foods may help manage and reduce these inflammatory responses, promoting a healthier back.

One of the best ways to target inflammation is by focusing on a variety of whole foods that are naturally rich in antioxidants, healthy fats, and essential nutrients. Let's take a closer look at some of the key anti-inflammatory foods to include in your diet:

1. Fatty Fish

Fatty fish like salmon, mackerel, and sardines are rich in omega-3 fatty acids. Omega-3s are known for their anti-inflammatory properties, as they help reduce inflammation in the body. Studies have shown that regular consumption of omega-3s can decrease the production of inflammatory markers and help with conditions like back pain. Aim for at least two servings of fatty fish per week to experience these benefits.

2. Berries

Berries such as blueberries, strawberries, raspberries, and blackberries are packed with antioxidants, especially anthocyanins, which have powerful anti-inflammatory effects. These compounds help reduce oxidative stress in the body, which contributes to inflammation. Adding a handful of berries to your daily routine, as well as in smoothies, on oatmeal, or as a snack.

3. Turmeric

Turmeric, specifically the compound curcumin, is another powerful anti-inflammatory food. Curcumin has been shown to reduce inflammation and relieve pain, making it an excellent addition to your diet if you're struggling with back pain. You can add turmeric to soups, stews, or smoothies, or drink it as part of a turmeric latte. For maximum absorption, pair turmeric with black pepper.

4. Leafy Greens

Dark, leafy greens like spinach, kale, and Swiss chard are rich in vitamins and minerals, including magnesium, which plays a key role in muscle function. Magnesium helps relax muscles and can reduce muscle spasms that often contribute to back pain. Leafy greens also provide antioxidants that help combat inflammation, making them essential for back health.

5. Nuts and Seeds

Nuts and seeds, particularly walnuts, almonds, and chia seeds, are good sources of healthy fats, fiber, and protein. These healthy fats, especially omega-3 fatty acids, can help lower inflammation. Walnuts, for example, have been shown to help decrease inflammatory markers in the body.

6. Olive Oil

Extra virgin olive oil is a staple of the Mediterranean diet, which is known for its anti-inflammatory benefits. Olive oil contains oleocanthal, a compound that has been shown to reduce inflammation in a similar way to ibuprofen. It's best to use olive oil as your primary cooking oil or drizzle it over salads, vegetables, or grains.

7. Ginger

Ginger is another natural anti-inflammatory food with a long history of use for treating pain and inflammation. It can help with reducing muscle pain and stiffness in the back. You can consume ginger in many forms, such as fresh ginger tea, smoothies, or as a spice in cooking.

8. Green Tea

Green tea is packed with polyphenols, which are potent antioxidants that can reduce inflammation. Drinking one or two cups of green tea daily can help manage chronic inflammation and promote overall health. It's also a good choice for hydration, which is important for muscle function and pain relief.

9. Tomatoes

Tomatoes are rich in lycopene, an antioxidant that helps reduce inflammation and pain, particularly in conditions like arthritis. Lycopene has been shown to reduce inflammation in the back and other parts of the body. Eating tomatoes in their raw form or as part of sauces can be a flavorful way to include them in your diet.

Strategic Suggestions

Incorporating these anti-inflammatory foods into your daily diet can be a game-changer for back health. Start by adding a few of these options to your meals and gradually increase your intake over time. Along with exercise and proper posture, a balanced diet rich in anti-inflammatory foods can help reduce pain and discomfort, allowing you to feel better and move more freely.

The Importance of Calcium and Vitamin D for Bone Health

Maintaining strong, healthy bones is essential for overall back health. Calcium and vitamin D are two of the most important nutrients for ensuring that your bones stay strong and resilient. A deficiency in these nutrients can lead to weakened bones, which can exacerbate back pain and increase your risk of injury.

The spine is made up of bones, discs, muscles, and ligaments that all work together to support your body. However, if your bones become brittle or weak, they can lead to conditions such as osteopenia or osteoporosis, which can cause pain, fractures, or even spinal deformities. Calcium and vitamin D play critical roles in the health of your bones, and making sure you get enough of both can help keep your back strong and support your overall posture.

The Role of Calcium in Bone Health

Calcium is the most abundant mineral in the body, and about 99% of it is stored in your bones and teeth. It plays a vital role in bone formation and strength. Calcium is also necessary for muscle function, nerve transmission, and blood clotting. When your body doesn't get enough calcium, it may begin to pull calcium from your bones, making them weaker over time.

For your back to stay strong and free of pain, it's essential to get an adequate amount of calcium. This will help maintain the integrity of the bones in your spine and prevent them from becoming fragile or brittle.

Good dietary sources of calcium include:

- Dairy products such as milk, yogurt, and cheese
- Leafy greens like kale, spinach, and collard greens
- Fortified plant-based milk (e.g., almond or soy milk)
- Tofu and fortified cereals
- Canned fish with soft bones, like sardines or salmon

If you are lactose intolerant or follow a plant-based diet, it's especially important to make sure you are consuming enough calcium from these alternative sources or consider supplementation if necessary. Generally, adults need around 1,000 mg of calcium daily, with a higher amount recommended for older adults (1,200 mg for women over 50 and men over 70).

The Role of Vitamin D in Bone Health

Vitamin D is essential for calcium absorption. Without vitamin D, your body cannot effectively absorb calcium from the foods you eat. It also helps regulate calcium levels in your blood and supports bone growth and remodeling. Vitamin D plays a crucial role in the prevention of bone disorders such as osteoporosis, which leads to weak, brittle bones and can cause back pain due to vertebral fractures.

Vitamin D is unique because it is produced in your skin when exposed to sunlight. However, in colder climates or during the winter months when sunlight exposure is limited, it can be harder for your body to produce enough vitamin D naturally. Therefore, it's important to consume vitamin D through food or supplements to ensure you are getting enough.

Vitamin D-rich foods include:

- Fatty fish like salmon, mackerel, and tuna
- Egg yolks
- Fortified foods like milk, orange juice, and cereals
- Mushrooms (especially those exposed to UV light)

The recommended daily amount of vitamin D varies based on age, with adults typically requiring 600 to 800 IU per day. However, older adults, those with limited sun exposure, or individuals with certain health conditions may need more. It is always advisable to talk to your doctor about vitamin D supplementation, as excessive intake can have negative effects.

How Calcium and Vitamin D Work Together

The relationship between calcium and vitamin D is vital for optimal bone health. Vitamin D enhances calcium absorption in the gut, ensuring that the calcium you consume reaches your bones. Without enough vitamin D, the body may not absorb enough calcium, even if your diet is rich in calcium. This can lead to weaker bones and an increased risk of fractures, which can directly affect your back health.

For example, a deficiency in either calcium or vitamin D can cause conditions such as osteopenia (a condition where bones become weaker than normal) and osteoporosis, both of which increase the likelihood of back pain and injuries, especially in the spine.

The Connection Between Bone Health and Back Pain

When your bones, including the vertebrae of the spine, become weakened, they may begin to compress or even fracture. This can lead to chronic pain, reduced mobility, and difficulty in everyday activities. Ensuring proper intake of calcium and vitamin D will help you maintain strong, healthy bones that support the spine and prevent such issues.

In addition to taking calcium and vitamin D, it's also important to maintain a well-rounded lifestyle that includes weight-bearing exercises to stimulate bone strength and improve posture. Pairing a strong nutritional foundation with regular physical activity will enhance the health of your back and decrease the chances of bone loss.

Strategic Suggestions

Incorporating enough calcium and vitamin D into your daily diet can make a huge difference for your back health. Ensure that you are giving your bones the proper nutrients they need, so you can improve strength, reduce pain, and enhance overall function. Remember to combine these nutrients with other strategies, such as exercise, proper posture, and stretching, for the best back health results.

Hydration: The Key to Muscle Function

Hydration is a crucial but often overlooked component of maintaining overall health and supporting your back. Water is not only vital for your organs and metabolism but also plays a major role in muscle function, including those muscles that support your spine. Without proper hydration, your muscles can become stiff, fatigued, and more prone to injury, leading to potential back pain.

We all know that drinking enough water is important for overall health, but did you know that staying properly hydrated can directly impact your back health? Your muscles are largely composed of water, and staying hydrated ensures that they can work properly. Hydration helps maintain muscle elasticity, reduce cramping, and prevent injuries, which are all key in managing and preventing back pain.

How Hydration Affects Muscle Function

Water makes up a large portion of your muscle cells, and it is essential for their function. Proper hydration helps muscles contract and relax efficiently, reducing the likelihood of muscle fatigue or strain. Dehydrated muscles are more likely to become stiff and tight, which can increase the risk of muscle spasms or pulls. These tight muscles can affect your posture, leading to misalignments in the spine that contribute to back pain.

When your muscles are well-hydrated, they are able to maintain their flexibility and strength. This is especially important for the muscles that support your back, including the muscles of your lower back, hips, and abdomen. These muscles need to be strong and flexible to maintain good posture and provide the necessary support for your spine throughout the day. If they are dehydrated and stiff, they are less capable of providing the support your back needs, making you more susceptible to pain and injury.

The Role of Hydration in Preventing Back Pain

Dehydration can contribute to back pain in a few key ways. First, when muscles are dehydrated, they can become tight and inflexible. This can lead to poor posture, which in turn puts additional stress on the spine and surrounding muscles. Poor posture is a common cause of chronic back pain because it puts strain on the muscles and ligaments of the back.

Additionally, dehydration can lead to muscle cramps and spasms, which can cause sudden, sharp pain in the back. These spasms occur when the muscles become involuntarily contracted due to a lack of water and other nutrients. This is especially common after prolonged physical activity or exercise when your body is losing water through sweat. Dehydration can also decrease the body's ability to repair muscle tissue after a workout, leading to longer recovery times and potential discomfort.

For your back to remain healthy, it's essential that you keep your muscles well-hydrated. This not only helps your muscles stay strong and flexible but also helps prevent the types of muscle spasms, cramps, and fatigue that often lead to back pain.

How Much Water Should You Drink?

The amount of water you need depends on your body size, level of activity, and climate. However, a good rule of thumb is to aim for about 8 cups (64 ounces) of water a day. If you are physically active or live in a hot climate, you may need more. For instance, if you're doing intense physical activity, you should drink additional water to replace the fluids lost through sweat.

To make sure you're getting enough, listen to your body. Thirst is an obvious indicator that you need water, but also pay attention to the color of your urine. If it's light yellow, you're well-hydrated. Dark yellow or amber-colored urine could indicate dehydration.

Hydration and Inflammation

In addition to helping muscles function properly, staying hydrated also supports your body's ability to manage inflammation. Chronic inflammation in the muscles and joints can lead to long-term back pain. When you are dehydrated, your body is less efficient at flushing out toxins and managing inflammation, which can increase discomfort.

Drinking enough water helps reduce the effects of inflammation and ensures that nutrients are delivered to the muscles more efficiently, which can assist in recovery and pain relief. Stay hydrated to help your body cope with inflammation better, potentially easing back pain and promoting a faster recovery after physical activity.

Hydration and Disc Health

The discs in your spine, which act as cushions between your vertebrae, also depend on hydration to maintain their integrity. These discs are made up of a gel-like substance that requires water to keep its shape and absorb shocks. If you're dehydrated, your discs can lose their ability to absorb pressure, which can lead to pain and increased risk of disc injuries. Proper hydration helps maintain disc health, ensuring that they can continue to protect the spine and prevent pain.

Tips for Staying Hydrated

Here are some tips to help you stay hydrated throughout the day:

1. Start your day with water

Drinking a glass of water as soon as you wake up can help kickstart your hydration.

2. Carry a water bottle

Keep a water bottle with you to remind yourself to drink throughout the day.

3. Add flavor

If you struggle with plain water, try adding a slice of lemon or cucumber for a refreshing taste.

4. Eat water-rich foods

Fruits and vegetables like cucumbers, watermelon, and oranges are full of water and can help contribute to your hydration.

Strategic Suggestions

Remember that hydration plays a critical role in maintaining muscle function and preventing back pain. Ensuring that your muscles are well-hydrated can improve flexibility, reduce muscle cramps, and support overall spinal health. Make hydration a regular part of your routine and pair it with proper exercise and nutrition for optimal back health.

Chapter 10: Putting It All Together

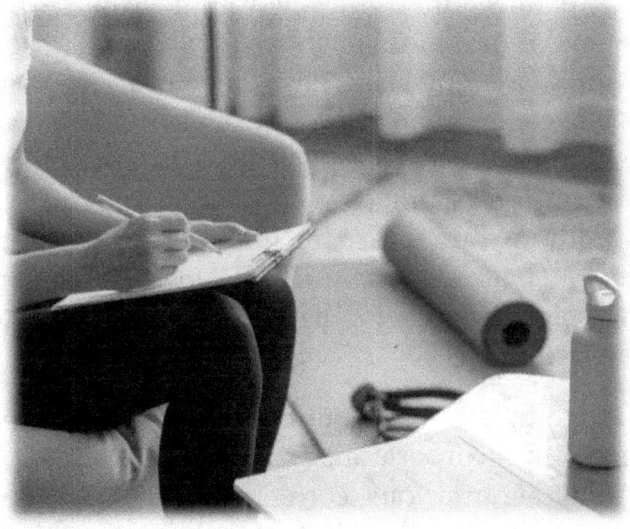

Putting it all together involves combining exercise, proper nutrition, and healthy habits to create a balanced approach to back health. This holistic strategy is key for strengthening muscles, improving posture, and preventing pain, ensuring long-term support and mobility for your back, while promoting overall well-being and function.

Designing a Weekly Routine for Back Pain Relief

A well-structured weekly routine can be an essential part of managing and alleviating back pain. Creating a consistent routine that includes a combination of exercises, stretches, and recovery periods will help to strengthen your muscles, improve flexibility, and reduce strain on your spine. It's important to keep in mind that back pain relief doesn't happen overnight, so developing a plan you can follow consistently is key to long-term improvement.

Designing a weekly routine for back pain relief involves incorporating exercises that focus on strengthening your core, improving posture, and enhancing flexibility. A balanced routine, when followed consistently, can provide significant relief from pain and prevent future discomfort. This routine should include a mix of strengthening and stretching exercises.

The foundation of any back pain relief routine is consistency. To maximize the effectiveness of your routine, it's essential to integrate exercises that target both the back and the surrounding muscle groups. Strengthening the core, glutes, and legs can provide support for the spine, while improving flexibility can help reduce muscle tightness and tension.

1. Strengthening Exercises

Core and Back Focus A strong core is vital for supporting your back. Core exercises, such as isometric planks and glute bridges, should be performed several times a week to target the muscles that help stabilize the spine. Planks, for instance, engage the abdominals, lower back, and even the shoulders, helping you develop a balanced foundation. Start with basic plank holds, working up to advanced variations as your strength increases.

In addition to core exercises, you should focus on strengthening your lower back. Incorporating exercises like the bird-dog hold, which strengthens the core while also stabilizing the back, can be highly beneficial. You can also add resistance training with exercises like the wall squat hold to work your quads and glutes, which help support the spine and reduce pressure on the lower back.

2. Stretching for Flexibility

Flexibility plays a huge role in maintaining a healthy back. Tight muscles can contribute to back pain, especially in areas like the hamstrings and hip flexors. Regular stretching should be included in your weekly routine to improve the flexibility of these muscles and reduce tension in your back. You can start with stretches like the cat-cow stretch, which gently mobilizes your spine, or the seated forward fold, which targets the hamstrings and lower back.

Other stretches, like the hip flexor stretch, will help lengthen the muscles around the pelvis and lower back. Include these stretches on a regular basis, so you can improve your overall mobility, which will alleviate stress on the spine.

3. Frequency and Progression

To create a successful weekly routine, you should aim to perform these exercises 3-4 times a week. This frequency allows you to strengthen and stretch your muscles while providing sufficient recovery time. Begin with lower intensity and gradually increase the duration or difficulty of the exercises as your body adapts.

For instance, if you're starting with planks, begin by holding the position for 20-30 seconds. As you get stronger, increase the duration to 45 seconds or 1 minute. Similarly, if you're doing wall sits, start with a 30-second hold and work up to 1 minute. Progression is key to continuing to challenge your muscles and promote growth.

Additionally, it's crucial to mix up the exercises in your routine to avoid overloading any single muscle group. You can alternate between core-focused exercises, lower body strengthening, and stretching routines to maintain a balanced approach. For example, on one day, you might do planks, glute bridges, and stretches for the hamstrings. The next day, you could focus on lower back strengthening and flexibility exercises.

4. Rest and Recovery

While exercises are essential for relieving back pain, rest and recovery are equally important. Your muscles need time to repair and grow stronger after each workout, so it's important to incorporate rest days into your routine. Depending on the intensity of your exercises, you should aim for at least one or two days of rest each week.

Active rest days can also be beneficial. These days might include light walking or gentle yoga stretches to keep your body moving without putting too much strain on your muscles. Remember that proper sleep, hydration, and nutrition all contribute to your body's ability to recover and stay strong.

5. Customizing Your Routine

Not everyone's back pain is the same, so your routine should be tailored to your specific needs. For some, back pain may stem from poor posture, while for others, it could be due to muscle imbalances or a lack of flexibility. You may need to experiment with different exercises to determine what works best for you. A good approach is to start with the basics and, as your body adapts, gradually introduce more challenging exercises or variations.

If you're unsure about how to start or if you experience pain while exercising, it may be helpful to consult with a physical therapist or a fitness professional who can guide you through the process and provide personalized advice.

Strategic Suggestions

Once you've established a routine, be patient with the process. Progress may be gradual, but with consistency and proper attention to your body's needs, you'll start to notice improvement. Track your exercises, listen to your body, and be open to adjusting your routine as needed to achieve the best results.

Tracking Your Progress and Adjusting Your Routine

Tracking your progress is an essential part of staying on track with your back pain relief journey. It helps you understand what's working, what might need adjustment, and how far you've come. If you're doing isometric exercises, stretching, or strength-building movements, keeping track of your progress allows you to stay motivated and focused.

Tracking your progress is essential for ensuring that your routine is working effectively. It helps you identify areas that need improvement, keep yourself motivated, and prevent injury. Regularly assessing your progress can also help you adjust your exercises and intensity as your body adapts to the training.

1. Tracking Pain and Discomfort

The primary reason for engaging in an exercise routine for back pain is to reduce discomfort. One of the first steps in tracking progress is to monitor your pain levels. Start by rating your pain on a scale of 1 to 10 before and after each workout. Over time, you should notice a reduction in pain or discomfort after performing your exercises. If your pain level remains unchanged or worsens, it's essential to adjust your exercises or seek professional guidance.

Pay attention to how your back feels throughout the day after you've exercised. Some discomfort or mild soreness is normal, but sharp or intense pain indicates that you may need to make modifications to your routine. Record how your back feels after each session to see any trends. If you find that certain exercises are causing pain, modify them by reducing the intensity, duration, or frequency, or replace them with alternative movements.

2. Monitoring Flexibility and Mobility

As your back pain improves, you should notice increased flexibility and better mobility. Flexibility plays a significant role in relieving back pain, as tight muscles can pull on your spine and contribute to discomfort. To track flexibility, test yourself periodically with stretches that target your hamstrings, lower back, and hip flexors.

For example, you might test how far you can reach in a seated forward fold stretch. Start by measuring how far you can reach when you begin your routine, and then check in every few weeks to see if you can reach farther. Similarly, you can measure the range of motion in your spine using stretches like the cat-cow stretch. Keep a journal of your flexibility improvements to celebrate your progress.

3. Tracking Strength and Endurance

Strengthening the muscles around your back, core, and legs plays a huge part in reducing back pain. It's important to track your strength improvements over time to ensure that your muscles are becoming stronger and better able to support your spine.

To track strength, start by noting how long you can hold an exercise like a plank or wall squat. As you continue practicing, aim to hold the position for longer or increase the number of repetitions you can do. For example, if you start with holding a plank for 20 seconds, gradually aim for 30, 45, or even 60 seconds. As you build endurance, you should also notice that your muscles fatigue less quickly.

You can also track progress by adjusting the intensity of the exercises. For example, if you're doing a wall squat, you can increase the time you hold the position or add more sets. Another way to increase difficulty is by adding variations, such as progressing from a basic plank to a side plank, or incorporating leg lifts into your bridge holds.

4. Adjusting Your Routine Based on Progress

As you track your progress, you'll notice areas of improvement and others that might need more attention. This is when adjustments to your routine become necessary. If you've become stronger and more flexible, you can increase the intensity of your exercises, add new movements, or increase the duration of holds. If you feel that some exercises are causing too much strain or pain, it's time to adjust them.

The key to adjusting your routine is to listen to your body. Start slowly and gradually increase the difficulty to avoid overstraining your muscles. You don't have to make drastic changes to see progress—small tweaks to your routine can make a big difference. For example, if a certain stretch no longer feels challenging, you might try holding it for a longer duration, or if a strength exercise becomes easy, add in a more advanced variation to increase the challenge.

As your strength, flexibility, and endurance improve, it's important to track your goals. Set short-term and long-term goals based on where you want to be. For example, a short-term goal might be to increase your plank hold from 20 to 30 seconds. A long-term goal could be to reach a certain level of flexibility in a hamstring stretch. Breaking down your progress into smaller, manageable goals keeps you motivated and gives you clear benchmarks for success.

5. Keeping a Journal or Log

A helpful way to track your progress is by keeping a fitness journal or log. Each day or week, jot down the exercises you performed, the duration of each hold, the number of sets or repetitions, and any notes about how you felt before, during, or after the session. This can be an effective way to reflect on how your body is responding to the routine and help you see patterns over time. If you feel like your progress is stagnating, your journal can help you pinpoint areas to adjust or challenges to focus on.

Strategic Suggestions

Tracking your progress helps you stay engaged with your routine and provides valuable feedback. Record pain levels, flexibility, strength, and endurance, so you can make informed adjustments to your exercises. Keep a journal to reflect on your progress and celebrate your improvements as you work toward a stronger, pain-free back.

When to Seek Professional Help

While an effective isometric exercise routine can make a significant difference in managing and alleviating back pain, there may be times when professional guidance is necessary. Knowing when to seek professional help can ensure your back health improves in a safe and effective manner. It's important to recognize when your back pain may need more attention than what an exercise routine alone can provide. If you find that your pain isn't improving or gets worse, seeking professional help from a healthcare provider can provide you with tailored treatment options and support.

1. Pain Persists Despite Regular Exercise

If you've been consistent with your isometric exercises, such as planks, glute bridges, and wall squats, yet you continue to experience pain or discomfort, it might be time to seek professional help. Sometimes pain can persist due to the underlying cause of the problem, such as a herniated disc, muscle imbalances, or degenerative conditions. If you have been diligent with your routine and haven't seen improvement, a healthcare provider can help determine if your pain stems from an issue that needs medical intervention, such as physical therapy, chiropractic care, or even imaging studies like X-rays or MRIs.

2. Increased Pain or New Symptoms

While mild soreness is common during exercise, experiencing new or increasing pain is a red flag. If your pain worsens during or after a workout, or you start feeling new symptoms such as numbness, tingling, weakness in your legs, or sharp pain radiating down your spine, it's critical to seek professional guidance. These could indicate that there's a more serious issue at play, such as nerve compression or other neurological conditions. In such cases, seeking medical help can help ensure that you receive the correct diagnosis and treatment plan.

3. Inability to Perform Basic Movements

If you find yourself unable to perform basic movements such as bending, standing, or walking without pain, it may be time to consult a professional. Difficulty moving freely is not only a sign that the issue might be more serious but also that your body may need more focused attention. A healthcare provider can guide you on how to move safely and prevent further injury, and can also recommend more advanced treatments like physical therapy or custom exercises to address your specific concerns.

4. Underlying Health Conditions

If you have pre-existing medical conditions such as arthritis, osteoporosis, scoliosis, or other spinal disorders, these can sometimes complicate back pain. In such cases, exercises and stretches may need to be tailored to your individual needs. A physical therapist or other healthcare professional can provide you with a customized exercise plan that takes your unique condition into account and helps avoid exacerbating the problem. They may also offer treatments like manual therapy or specialized stretches that are not only safe but more effective for your specific needs.

5. Emotional or Psychological Factors

Sometimes, the persistence of back pain can be linked to emotional and psychological factors, such as stress, anxiety, or depression. These can affect how your body perceives and responds to pain. If you notice that your pain seems to be influenced by your mood or stress levels, seeking the help of a professional who can address these underlying factors might be helpful. A mental health professional or therapist can help you manage stress and anxiety that might be making your back pain worse.

6. Personalized Assessment and Treatment

One of the best reasons to consult a professional is for a personalized assessment. Physical therapists, chiropractors, or orthopedic doctors are experts in evaluating back pain and offering individualized treatment plans that go beyond general exercise advice. They can evaluate your posture, muscle imbalances, spinal alignment, and joint mobility. Once they understand the full scope of the issue, they can design a comprehensive treatment plan that includes hands-on therapy, stretching techniques, strengthening exercises, or other interventions to address your pain.

Physical therapists, for example, can work with you one-on-one to guide you through corrective exercises and teach you the proper form and techniques to improve mobility and strength safely. They may also use modalities like heat or cold therapy, ultrasound therapy, or electrical stimulation to manage pain and promote healing.

7. Preventing Further Injury

In some cases, improper form or overexertion can lead to injury. If you find yourself constantly battling the same muscle strains, joint discomfort, or pain after workouts, a professional can help you identify and correct issues with your technique. This can prevent further injury and ensure that your exercise routine remains safe and effective. They can also help you understand your body's limits, ensuring that you don't push yourself too hard too soon, which could otherwise hinder your recovery.

8. Surgery and Medical Interventions

In rare cases, if non-invasive treatments like exercise, physical therapy, and lifestyle changes aren't sufficient, a medical professional may recommend surgery or more advanced procedures to treat serious conditions such as herniated discs, severe nerve compression, or fractures. While this is not common, knowing when surgery or other interventions might be needed is important for long-term back health. If your back pain is caused by something structural or degenerative, seeking medical advice will guide you toward the best course of action.

Strategic Suggestions

Knowing when to seek professional help is key to ensuring that your back pain doesn't worsen or lead to further complications. If your pain persists, increases, or interferes with your daily life, don't hesitate to consult with a healthcare provider. They can offer targeted solutions and provide the best care for your condition.

Chapter 11: Maintaining Long Term Back Health

Maintaining long-term back health involves consistent care through exercise, proper posture, and healthy lifestyle choices. This approach is essential for preventing pain, improving mobility, and keeping the spine strong. Commit to these habits to ensure lasting support for your back and reduce the risk of future discomfort or injury.

Preventing Future Back Pain

Preventing future back pain is crucial to maintaining a healthy, active lifestyle. If you've experienced back pain in the past or are working to prevent it from happening, it's important to take proactive steps. While exercises and stretches are essential, lifestyle choices such as posture, hydration, and regular activity can make all the difference. Implementing a combination of preventative practices will not only keep your spine healthy but also help you live pain-free.

One of the most important aspects of preventing future back pain is focusing on maintaining strong, flexible muscles around the spine. Regular isometric exercises, such as those you've learned in this book, help to build a solid foundation. These exercises engage the core, back, and lower body muscles, providing support for your spine. You'll need to strengthen these muscles to reduce the strain on your back, making it less likely that you'll experience pain or discomfort in the future.

It's also essential to incorporate stretching into your routine to maintain flexibility. Tight muscles, especially in the lower back, hamstrings, and hips, can contribute to back pain. Stretching these areas regularly helps to maintain mobility, reduce muscle tension, and prevent stiffness. Flexibility exercises such as the Cat-Cow stretch, forward folds, and hip stretches can go a long way in keeping your back healthy.

Another key factor in preventing future back pain is proper posture. How you sit, stand, and move throughout the day impacts the health of your spine. For example, sitting for long periods with poor posture can lead to muscle imbalances, spinal misalignment, and unnecessary strain on your back. It's important to sit with your feet flat on the floor, keeping your knees at a 90-degree angle. Try to avoid slouching, as this places excessive pressure on the lower back. If you work at a desk, make sure your workstation is ergonomically friendly, and take breaks to stand and stretch.

Standing posture is just as important. When you stand, make sure your weight is evenly distributed between both feet, and avoid locking your knees. Engaging your core muscles helps support your lower back and prevents strain. Keep your shoulders relaxed but back, and avoid leaning forward or backward. Proper alignment reduces the risk of developing back pain over time.

Incorporating regular physical activity into your routine is another powerful way to prevent back pain. While targeted exercises like those discussed earlier are important, staying active overall is key. Activities such as walking, swimming, or cycling keep your body moving and promote circulation, which helps nourish the discs in your spine and keeps your muscles and ligaments strong.

When lifting objects, use proper lifting techniques to protect your back. Instead of bending over at the waist, bend at your knees, squat down, and keep the object close to your body. Engaging your core and using your legs to lift rather than your back reduces strain and minimizes the risk of injury. Lifting with your back can lead to muscle strains or more serious injuries, so be mindful of your movements.

In addition to exercise and posture, nutrition plays a crucial role in back health. A balanced diet rich in anti-inflammatory foods, such as leafy greens, fatty fish, and nuts, can help manage any inflammation in your body that could contribute to back pain. Staying hydrated is also essential, as it helps keep the discs in your spine lubricated, promoting their proper function and reducing the risk of injury.

Another important practice in preventing future back pain is to manage stress. Stress can contribute to muscle tension, particularly in the back and neck areas. Incorporating stress-relieving practices like deep breathing, yoga, or meditation into your routine can reduce the impact of stress on your body. Managing your stress levels helps keep your muscles relaxed and your back pain-free.

It's essential to remember that prevention is an ongoing commitment. Consistency in exercise, posture, nutrition, and stress management is key. While you may not be able to control all the factors that affect your back health, you can take responsibility for the habits and practices that will help you feel your best and protect your spine.

Strategic Suggestions

To ensure long-term back health, create a daily or weekly routine that includes core strengthening, flexibility exercises, and posture checks. Continue to make mindful choices about how you move, sit, and stand throughout the day. Lastly, listen to your body and adjust your routine as needed to avoid any strain or discomfort.

Staying Consistent with Your Exercises

Staying consistent with your exercises is one of the most effective ways to prevent and manage back pain. Consistency helps to build strength, flexibility, and muscle memory, all of which are essential in supporting your spine and maintaining back health. If you've already experienced back pain, developing a consistent routine will also help reduce the likelihood of it returning. However, the key is to make these exercises a regular part of your day rather than treating them as temporary fixes. Here's how you can stay consistent and turn your exercise routine into a lifelong habit.

One of the biggest obstacles to staying consistent with exercises is finding the motivation to stick with it. The good news is that once you experience the benefits of consistent exercise—such as reduced pain, better posture, and increased energy—it becomes easier to stay on track. Start by setting clear, achievable goals. This could mean committing to a certain number of days per week to perform your exercises, or aiming for a specific duration of time each session. Keep your goals realistic and celebrate small victories along the way.

Having a set routine is another important factor. Consistency thrives on structure, so scheduling your exercises at the same time each day or week helps establish a habit. For instance, you might choose to do your back exercises every morning before breakfast or right before bed to wind down. The more you make it part of your daily schedule, the less likely you'll be to skip or forget it.

Another way to stay consistent is by creating a workout space that's inviting and free of distractions, like a corner of your living room, a designated home gym, or even a spot outside. Make sure the area is comfortable and accessible. Having a consistent space to do your exercises makes the process feel easier and more natural. You don't need fancy equipment—just a mat or cushion and some open space to get started.

Tracking your progress is also a great motivator. Keep a simple log of the exercises you do, the number of sets, and how you feel afterward. Noticing improvements, such as a reduction in pain, increased flexibility, or more strength, will help you stay motivated and remind you why you're putting in the effort. Tracking progress also gives you the chance to make adjustments when necessary. For example, if you notice certain exercises are helping more than others, you can emphasize them in your routine.

To ensure you stay on track, consider incorporating variety into your exercises. Doing the same routine every day can become monotonous, which might lead to burnout. Mix up the isometric exercises, stretches, and movements you're doing to keep things interesting. You could also try new variations of the exercises you're already familiar with, like changing your plank position or adding weights to your glute bridges. This will keep your routine fresh and give your muscles different challenges to adapt to.

Social support can also be a big help in staying consistent. Consider enlisting a friend or family member to join you in your exercise routine. This can make it more enjoyable and keep you accountable. If working out with someone isn't an option, consider joining online communities or forums where people share tips, experiences, and progress updates. Being part of a group that encourages each other can boost motivation and help you stay on track.

Remember to listen to your body as you stay consistent with your exercises. If you're feeling pain (not just discomfort), it's important to stop and reassess. Overdoing it can lead to injury, so make sure to take rest days when needed and not push yourself too hard.

Recovery is just as important as the exercises themselves.

If you ever miss a day or two, don't get discouraged. Life happens, and it's easy to fall off track. The important thing is to get back into your routine as soon as possible. Being kind to yourself when things don't go perfectly can make it easier to stay consistent in the long run.

Strategic Suggestions

To maintain consistency with your exercises, set achievable goals, create a structured routine, and track your progress. Keep your exercise environment welcoming and varied, and consider involving a friend for motivation. Listen to your body, stay flexible, and remember that persistence will pay off in the long run.

Final Tips for a Healthy Spine

Maintaining a healthy spine isn't just about exercises; it's also about making mindful choices throughout your daily life. Your back health relies on a combination of good habits, proper posture, appropriate physical activity, and attention to your body's needs. In this section, we'll discuss some final tips for ensuring your spine stays in top shape, helping you stay free from back pain and discomfort for the long haul.

1. Prioritize Posture

Good posture plays a critical role in maintaining back health. While sitting, standing, or walking, your spine needs to stay aligned to prevent strain and tension. Start by paying attention to how you sit throughout the day. If you're sitting at a desk, make sure your chair supports your lower back, and your feet are flat on the floor. Your knees should be at a 90-degree angle, and your shoulders should be relaxed, not hunched forward. When standing, avoid locking your knees and try to distribute your weight evenly between both feet. This will help reduce pressure on your spine.

When walking, try to maintain a neutral spine position with your head held high and your shoulders back. Avoid slouching or leaning forward, as this can put unnecessary stress on your back. If you tend to carry heavy bags, switch them from one side to the other to prevent uneven pressure on your spine.

2. Regular Movement is Key

While exercises like planks, bridges, and stretches are essential for strengthening your back, it's also important to avoid staying in one position for too long. Prolonged sitting or standing can cause stiffness and tightness in your spine, so make it a habit to move throughout the day. If you work at a desk, set a timer to remind yourself to stand up and stretch every 30 minutes. Even if it's just for a minute or two, moving around helps keep your spine limber and reduces the risk of back pain.

Simple movements, such as standing and walking around, can keep your muscles engaged and your back aligned. If possible, try incorporating activities like walking, cycling, or swimming into your routine, as these low-impact exercises can improve spinal flexibility and strength.

3. Maintain a Healthy Weight

Carrying excess weight, especially around the abdomen, can put added stress on your lower back. The extra weight pulls your pelvis forward, causing your spine to curve unnaturally, which can lead to pain and discomfort. Eating a balanced diet, staying active, and maintaining a healthy weight are all important factors in reducing the strain on your back.

Consider adopting a diet rich in anti-inflammatory foods, including fruits, vegetables, lean proteins, and whole grains. These foods can help prevent inflammation, which is often a cause of back pain. Staying hydrated is just as important, as it keeps the discs in your spine hydrated and functioning properly.

4. Practice Stress Management

Stress doesn't just affect your mind—it can also affect your body, especially your back. When you're stressed, your muscles tend to tighten, which can lead to back stiffness and pain. Finding ways to manage stress, such as practicing mindfulness, meditation, deep breathing exercises, or even simple relaxation techniques, can be beneficial for your spine.

Make sure you're taking time each day to unwind and relax. such as through deep breathing, a warm bath, or listening to calming music. These activities can help relieve tension in your back and promote overall well-being.

5. Be Mindful of Lifting Techniques

Proper lifting techniques are essential for protecting your back. No matter if you're lifting groceries, children, or other heavy objects, always bend your knees and use your legs to lift, not your back. Keep the object close to your body and avoid twisting while lifting. If something is too heavy, ask for help or use assistive devices like carts or lifting straps.

6. Stay Hydrated

Hydration is often overlooked when it comes to back health, but it plays an important role. Your spinal discs are made of cartilage, and they need water to stay flexible and absorb shock. Dehydration can cause your discs to lose their cushioning ability, leading to increased pressure on your spine. Drink plenty of water throughout the day to keep your body hydrated and support the health of your spine.

7. Sleep Support

Your spine needs proper support while you sleep to recover from the day's activities. Make sure your mattress is firm enough to support your spine's natural curvature. Avoid sleeping on your stomach, as this position can strain your neck and lower back. Instead, try sleeping on your back with a pillow under your knees or on your side with a pillow between your knees to help maintain spinal alignment.

8. Listen to Your Body

Finally, one of the most important tips for a healthy spine is to listen to your body. If you start feeling discomfort or pain in your back, take a break and assess what might be causing it. Sometimes, all it takes is a small adjustment in posture or a change in activity to relieve the pressure. If pain persists, don't hesitate to consult a healthcare professional to get guidance on how to address the issue.

Strategic Suggestions

Prioritize good posture, incorporating regular movement, manage stress, and adopt healthy lifestyle habits, so you can ensure long-term back health. Always be mindful of your body's signals and make necessary adjustments to prevent strain. Stay consistent with exercises and make adjustments as needed to support a strong and healthy spine.

Conclusion

By now, you've gained valuable tools to address back pain, strengthen your body, and improve your overall quality of life. This book has guided you through the science behind isometric exercises, step-by-step routines, and practical advice to build a healthier, pain-free back. With these techniques, you're equipped to take charge of your well-being and move confidently into a future with less discomfort and more freedom.

To make the most of what you've learned, remember to be consistent with your exercises and listen to your body. Progress may take time, but every step forward is a step toward lasting relief. Pair your workouts with good posture, proper hydration, and a balanced diet to amplify the benefits.

You've started a powerful journey to back health, and your efforts will pay off. Take pride in what you've achieved so far, and keep building on this foundation. If this book has helped you, consider sharing your experience through a review. Your feedback not only helps other readers discover these valuable methods but also supports the author in creating more helpful resources.

For further reading, explore other titles by the author, including guides on core strength, functional fitness, and nutrition for a pain-free life. Each book is crafted to complement your efforts and expand your understanding of holistic health and wellness.

As you wind down, keep this in mind: you are your greatest advocate for health and vitality. With the knowledge and techniques from this book, you hold the key to lasting back health. Take care of your body, stay consistent, and enjoy the strength and freedom you've worked to achieve.

www.ingramcontent.com/pod-product-compliance
Lightning Source LLC
Chambersburg PA
CBHW071021240526
45469CB00006BD/2023